Case Studies in

Erford

Community
Health
Nursing
Practice

A Problem-Based Learning Approach

D1296612

Juliann G. Sebastian, RN, PhD, CS
Assistant Dean for Advanced Practice Nursing and Associate Professor
College of Nursing
University of Kentucky
Lexington, Kentucky

Marcia Stanhope, RN, DSN, FAAN, c
Associate Dean and Professor
College of Nursing
University of Kentucky
Lexington, Kentucky

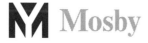 Mosby

St. Louis Baltimore Boston Carlsbad Chicago Minneapolis New York Philadelphia Portland
London Milan Sydney Tokyo Toronto

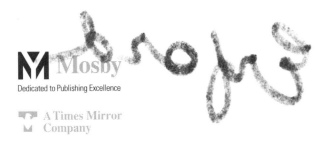

M Mosby
Dedicated to Publishing Excellence

A Times Mirror
Company

Publisher: Sally Schrefer
Executive Editor: June Thompson
Editor: Loren Wilson
Senior Developmental Editor: Linda Caldwell
Developmental Editor: Rae Robertson
Project Manager: Deborah L. Vogel
Production Editor: Ed Alderman
Designer: Bill Drone
Cover Designer: E. Rohne Rudder
Manufacturing Manager: Dave Graybill

Composition by Graphic World, Inc.
Printing/binding by Malloy Lithographing

Mosby, Inc.
11830 Westline Industrial Drive
St. Louis, Missouri 63146

International Standard Book Number 0-323-00260-9

98 99 00 01 02 / 9 8 7 6 5 4 3 2 1

Contributing Authors

Margaret "Peggy" Hickman, MSN, EdD

Associate Professor
College of Nursing and the University of Kentucky Center for
  Rural Health
University of Kentucky
Lexington, Kentucky

Marilyn Givens King, MN, DNSc

Associate Professor
College of Nursing and The University of Kentucky Center for
  Rural Health
University of Kentucky
Lexington, Kentucky

Special thanks to Dr. Ellen Hahn, Assistant Professor, University of Kentucky College of Nursing and Dr. Ruth Knollmueller, past coordinator for the College of Nursing at the University of Kentucky Center for Rural Health. These two individuals contributed their time and effort to the working groups which developed the initial cases. Special thanks to the students in NUR 620—Issues in Rural Health Delivery, for their contribution to the development of the rural health cases.

Partial support for the development of this manuscript was provided by the United States Public Health Service, DHHS, Health Resources and Services Administration, Division of Nursing, Grant ID#23-NU-01039, Principal Investigator, Marcia Stanhope.

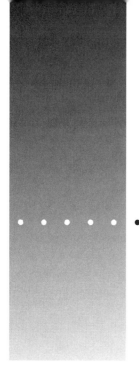

Foreword

Learning is contextual. If asked to recall the facts and concepts presented in a particular course taken several years ago, most of us would remember very few of the discrete bits of information that we had "learned." That is because learning occurs best in the context in which the information will be used.

The cases presented in this book provide opportunities for students to learn in "real" situations—situations that mimic real communities that the student will encounter in practice. Thus the new concepts, theories, and information encountered in this text will more likely be remembered and used in the future. In addition to acquiring and applying new knowledge, students who use these cases as a stimulus for learning will have the opportunity to develop their reasoning and study skills. The cases should bring a sense of reality and excitement to the learning process.

We are grateful to the case writers for sharing what they have learned by developing the cases presented in this book.

Phyllis P. Nash, EdD

Vice Chancellor for Academic and Student Affairs
A.B. Chandler Medical Center
University of Kentucky
Lexington, Kentucky

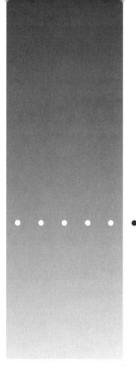

Preface

The cases in this book reflect the broad range of community health nursing practice opportunities available for professional nurses. The process of thinking through these cases, questioning current assumptions, and investigating existing learning issues will strengthen critical thinking and analysis skills. These skills are essential in the contemporary health care environment, contributing to the student's effectiveness as a professional and as a leader in providing community health nursing services that will improve health outcomes of clients, families, and communities.

It is our hope that these cases will stimulate continued learning about community health nursing and contribute to clinical expertise, thereby helping to solve some of the pressing health problems facing local communities.

Juliann G. Sebastian
Marcia Stanhope

Contents

Part I

Introduction to Problem-Based Learning

1 Critical Thinking in Community Health Nursing

Marcia Stanhope

Community health nursing is similar to all other clinical specialties in that it is a practice discipline with an identified client group. However, in community health the client is identified as a community or aggregate. The aggregate may be a family, a group of families, or a nonfamily group with similar needs. The community may be defined as a community of solution, a geographically defined community, or a community of targeted health problems. The clinical arena for the community health nurse thus varies with the type of client one may have at a given point. Education of the community health nurse and clinical specialist in public health requires the integration of a wide range of knowledge and experiences to address the needs of these clients, including content in epidemiology, biostatistics, program management and research methods, community development, nursing concepts/theories/interventions, delivery models, and policy development, to name a few.

To be able to integrate this array of knowledge and skills for appropriate problem assessment and interventions, the community health nurse and the clinical specialist must become critical thinkers and possess quality clinical decision-making skills. Whereas classroom lectures/seminars and structured clinical practica have been the mainstays of nursing education, critical thinking and clinical decision-making skills can best be developed by allowing the learner to explore and experience critical situations firsthand.

The development of these skills comes through discovery and self-definition of problems, a search for alternatives, a commitment to testing the proposed alternatives, carrying out the alternatives, and evaluating the results of one's actions (Joyce and Weil, 1986; Barrows and Feltovich, 1987). This approach to learning is best suited to the adult learner, who brings to the classroom a wealth of knowledge gained through past education and life and professional experiences.

However, the optimum educational benefit is facilitated by a teacher who can guide the exploration process so that the student is exposed to the complexities and types of problems that may be presented by clients. Such an approach allows active exploration, with the faculty member serving as a guide through this experience.

Problem-based learning is an approach to teaching and learning that allows for problem exploration. Fundamentally different from traditional educational methods such as lectures and seminars, it features problem-solving activities that encourage the application or use of acquired knowledge. Problem-based learning has several distinguishing characteristics, including:

- Learning based on reality and the contextual nature of practice
- Fostering critical thinking and the reasoning process
- Self-directed learning
- Traditional knowledge integration based on the situation under discussion in tutorial sessions (Townsend, 1990)

A variety of approaches exist for presenting problems in this manner; however, the case study method has been chosen for this text. The case study method (Barrows and Feltovich, 1987; Waterman and Butler, 1985) presents a concrete description of a situation relevant to professional practice, including pertinent facts and opinions as well as distracting information, for which the student must develop a solution using community-specific resources. The student is asked to assume a specific role in developing the solution. When an optimal alternative is put forth, the rationality of selecting that approach over competing approaches must be justified.

Throughout, the process of case analysis focuses on problems similar to those encountered in real clinical situations. This format encourages the development of critical-thinking and resource identification skills. Students will work together to identify group and individual strengths and plot the direction for the case analysis. Tutored group work helps in the development of group work skills, communication skills, and conflict resolution skills.

The student begins by identifying what is already known or believed to be true about the situation; then moves to set individual learning goals based on individual analysis of the case and the group discussion. In this way individual values, biases, beliefs, and assumptions are highlighted for validation or refutation. The faculty tutor can then involve the group in values clarification exercises.

Because the responsibility for learning is shifted and because time for study is protected, the student is encouraged to develop better study skills and become more self-directed. These are necessary skills for lifelong learning. Finally, problem-based learning helps develop self-assessment and evaluation skills, as well as group evaluation skills.

2 Problem-Based Learning for the Student

Margaret "Peggy" Hickman

This book of case studies is designed to be used in conjunction with planned group activities in the classroom under the guidance of a faculty facilitator. Each case is fictitious and was developed to represent the clinical issues in contemporary community health nursing practice. The book may be used by undergraduates in community health courses and graduate students in clinical specialist programs. The student will begin by working alone, then move to group discussions guided by the faculty facilitator.

A real-life clinical situation will serve as the starting point for using critical thinking skills to explore concepts in community health and nursing care. As in real life, the cases include some controversial ideas that students should identify and analyze. By becoming an active partner in the education process, the student can identify what information is needed to "solve" each case and pursue the answers through individual and group self-directed learning activities. This educational method is intended to help:

- Structure knowledge based in a clinical context
- Develop clinical reasoning skills
- Develop critical thinking skills
- Develop effective self-directed learning skills
- Develop effective interpersonal skills
- Develop skills in self-assessment and evaluation
- Develop skills in peer assessment and evaluation

CASE ANALYSIS

Before working with other students and the faculty facilitator to resolve the case problem, the student should:

- Read the case.
- List the concepts discussed in the case.
- After careful review, list what is known about the case.
- Identify what new information is needed to solve the problem or better understand the situation.
- Read references given on the topic or choose readings independently to learn what is not already known. A selection of references relevant to each case is provided at the end of the book.
- Contact a resource person(s) and discuss the case to validate existing knowledge about the problem.
- Share findings with a group of peers and the faculty facilitator.
- Together, evaluate the outcomes of the case.

GROUP ACTIVITIES

Each case includes a series of modules describing a clinical situation. Some cases describe situations occurring over a period of years, while others take place in much shorter time frames. The following format for problem-based learning sessions is recommended for use with each module.

Independent (Individual) Study Before Each Group Session

The student will:

- Read texts, journals, research reports, epidemiological reports, and other material that address identified learning issue(s).
- Explore additional education resources as needed.
- Consult with faculty as necessary.
- Practice skills being learned from the case in the clinical area.
- Compile data as needed to support hypotheses about the case.

Group Exploration of Case

The student will:

- Read the clinical case or situation aloud.
- Identify what is already known, based on prior and concurrent course work, clinical experience, and information revealed in the case.
- Identify nursing, epidemiologic, and other related concepts, problems, and issues in the case.
- Generate hypotheses.
- Identify additional data needed.
- Identify learning issues/needs.
- Identify/allocate tasks for the next group session (for example, assign each of the newly identified learning issues to group members who can discuss them at the next meeting).

Ground Rules

When the students come together as a group with the faculty facilitator, the problem-based teaching/learning method will be more effective if the following guidelines are followed:

- Everyone participates.
- Collaboration, rather than competition, is rewarded.
- No one is assumed to have knowledge specific to each case. The cases are designed to help learners identify and pursue new areas of inquiry.
- Each person is an active learner.
- Each member of the group is responsible for facilitating discussion and for identifying and pursuing individual and group learning needs.
- There are no inappropriate or "dumb" questions.

Subsequent Classes (Same Case)

The student will:

- Summarize findings/sources of information.
- Gradually eliminate data that are unrelated to the key concepts and issues in the case.
- Move to the next section of the case or to a new case.

Timing of Case

Students should:

- Complete each case within three class sessions.

3 Journaling as an Approach to Student Learning

Juliann G. Sebastian

The cases in this workbook will help the student analyze clinical situations in community health and learn more about the theoretical underpinnings of community health nursing interventions. One way to maximize this learning process is through the use of a journal to help identify what is being learned, question current assumptions, and analyze how learning today will influence work as a professional nurse in the future. Journaling has become a highly regarded strategy for enhancing critical thinking skills (Brookfield, 1995) and developing "reflective practitioners" (Schon, 1983), or clinicians who use a personal and professional value system as the basis for decision-making. This section of the workbook describes how to use a journal to learn through problem-based cases.

The purpose of problem-based learning is to enhance understanding through the integration of real-life examples, the sequential search for information, development of the meaning of that information in relation to clinical practice and professional values, and the strengthening of critical thinking skills.

Problem-based learning uses a thinking process known as "hypothetico-deductive reasoning" (Barrows, 1988) that mirrors the usual reasoning process used by expert clinicians. In this process, learners receive some information about a situation and begin to identify cues present in that information that suggest certain problems or issues that may be present or that could arise. The information is only a snapshot and not a full presentation of the sequence of events, because in real practice, one sees only small parts of a clinical scenario at any one time.

Learners are asked to identify what data are actually available in the portion of the scenario they are reading, and to differentiate data from hunches. Hunches about potential problems or issues are actually "provisional hypotheses" and need to be verified or discarded based on further data collection and testing of hypotheses. The process of data acquisition, analysis and testing, identification of additional data needed to rule in or rule out a provisional hypothesis, and eventual development of strategies for problem resolution is mirrored in a problem-based learning case.

In order to work through the cases in this workbook using the hypothetico-deductive reasoning process, the student should answer the following questions with each segment of a case (Nash, 1994; King, Sebastian, Stanhope, and Hickman, 1997):

1. ***What actual data or information do I have about this case?*** Test this point by reviewing the case to determine what really are data and what is an inference from the data. For example, a case study might report: "Sharon looked away and sighed." The data in that situation are strictly behavioral; i.e., that Sharon looked away and sighed. The data are not that "Sharon was discouraged" or "Sharon was angry" or "Sharon was tired." Each of these statements might represent a hunch, or a provisional hypothesis, about what is occurring. To validate one or more of these hypotheses, additional information is needed. Just as in real clinical situations, some of the data is unrelated to the issues of concern to the nurse. Part of the critical thinking process involves differentiating data that is relevant to the key problems or concerns from that which is irrelevant. This leads to the second question the student should ask.

2. ***What other data do I need to better understand this situation?*** In this case, one might conclude that someone should ask Sharon how she is feeling. It may be learned that Sharon's nursing job is being redesigned from one that is strictly hospital-based to one that includes home visits with recently discharged clients. Sharon could be worried about whether she has the skills necessary to provide community-based care to clients and families. Sharon's response either will help validate one of your provisional hypotheses or help develop a new hypothesis. It is important to identify all of the provisional, or working, hypotheses so the student can systematically determine which are valid.

3. ***What are my provisional hypotheses?*** This is another way of asking, "What might be going on in this situation?" It is helpful to develop a list of provisional hypotheses as they come to mind so they can systematically be tested to determine which, if any, is a valid representation of the situation. These hypotheses might be in the form of problem or need statements; or they might be in the form of if-then statements. For example, early in a case, one hypothesis might be, "Sharon is anxious about the change in her job because she feels unprepared for the new responsibilities." Another hypothesis might be, "*If* she is provided with educational opportunities to help her learn how to provide community-based care to clients and families, *then* she will not be as anxious and will be more likely to be effective in her new role." This last hypothesis might lead the student to question

whether inservice education, continuing education, or formal academic preparation are effective ways of learning new job skills and reducing anxiety. In that case, a learning issue has been identified.

4. *What learning issues have I identified in this case?* These are the areas which must be explored in order to be able to manage successfully in a similar situation. These areas will be investigated through the use of written materials, interviews with experts and consumers, and electronic resource searches of the Internet. Each chapter in Part II contains a list of suggested resources as a starting point. Printed references are listed at the end of the book. If a learning issue is identified for which no relevant references or resources are listed, begin to search by reviewing the professional literature.

Finally, at the end of each case, consider the following questions and record the answers in a journal. These questions (Driscoll, 1994) encourage the ongoing process of self-discovery and critical reflection:

1. *What?* What have I learned from this case? (Answering this question will help summarize all of the new concepts mastered while working through the learning issues.)
2. *So What?* What do these new ideas that I have learned mean to me as a professional nurse? Have I learned anything that changes my assumptions or strengthens my beliefs and values? What implications do these new ideas have for my role as a professional nurse? Will I function any differently as a result of my learning? If so, how?
3. *Now What?* How will I use what I have learned in other classes? How will I use this new learning and these new realizations about my beliefs, values, and assumptions in my future as a professional nurse? How will I use these new ideas to behave as a professional outside of my paid employment in the areas of political involvement, nursing in my neighborhood and community, or as a citizen within my community?

Part
II
Case Studies

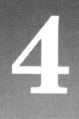

4 Practice Roles and Issues

Marcia Stanhope

It is widely understood that an effective health care system addresses quality, cost, access, and acceptability of care to all citizens. In recent years there has been a great deal of attention to health care reform. In actuality, this has been a debate on how medical care is organized, financed, and delivered. Little has been done to place more emphasis on prevention—a reform which could save lives, reduce chronic illness, improve the environment, and redirect money to arenas other than health care, such as education, leisure, retirement, and community development.

The need to focus attention on disease prevention, health promotion, and lifestyle factors—which together account for 50% of all unnecessary deaths in the United States—led to the development of a healthy public policy for the nation, Healthy People 2000. It identifies a comprehensive set of goals to address disease prevention and health promotion.

Because people do not always know how to maximize their health status, the challenge for community health nurse generalists and nurse clinical specialists is to be a catalyst for change. It is imperative that nurses be visionary in designing their roles and identifying practice arenas. To do this, nurses need to understand concepts and theories of public health and nursing practice; the changing health care delivery system; actual and potential roles and responsibilities of nurses and other health care providers; the importance of disease prevention and health promotion; the role of the consumer in health care; and the effects of planning, implementation, and evaluation of health care services.

The case studies in this chapter address (1) issues of professional development; (2) accessibility of health care and practice arrangements in the health care delivery system; (3) roles and functions of health care providers, the historical development of nursing, and the context of community health nursing practice; and (4) factors affecting health as well as the development of health policy and the politics of health promotion and disease prevention.

Case Study 4A, Charlene Bishop, emphasizes the historical development of the nurse's role in community health/public health and practice-related functions. The context of practice is explored as the nurse manager of a large community organization seeks to justify funding for advanced practice nurse positions, including community health clinical specialists and the community health nurse generalists who provide care to a population.

Case Study 4B, Mary, explores the needs of client populations and, through collaborative efforts, seeks to address access issues in the health care delivery system at county and regional levels.

Case Study 4C, Mrs. Beatty, provides an opportunity to analyze provider behaviors, educational and credentialing issues, and regulation of practice and ethical issues.

Finally, Case Study 4D, Alice McDermott, interweaves the determinants of health with strategies for health promotion and disease prevention. The role of politics is also explored as it relates to the development of health policy.

Resources

People Resources: Persons to interview to clarify case concepts

- Nurse legislators on politics
- Nurse lawyer on policy development
- Health department nurse consultant
- Community health nurse faculty
- Community health nurse (generalist, specialist, manager, case manager)

Electronic Resources: Office of Disease Prevention and Health Promotion (ODPHP) Web sites

ODPHP	http://odphp.osophs.dhhs.gov/
healthfinder™	http://www.healthfinder.gov/
Healthy People 2000	http://odphp.osophs.dhhs.gov/pubs/hp2000/
Healthy People 2010 Home Page	http://web.health.gov/healthypeople/
National Health Information Center	http://nhic-nt.health.org/
Partnerships Conference	http://odphp.osophs.dhhs.gov/confrnce/ partnr97/
Put Prevention Into Practice	http://www.dhhs.gov/PPIP

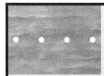 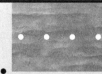

Case Study 4A • Part One
Charlene Bishop

Case Material

"We're just going to have to cut back in order to meet our budget," Bob Isaacs said. "Since most of our money is tied up in salaries, I think that is the place where the cutbacks will have to take place. I recommend that we eliminate some of these master of science in nursing (MSN) positions because I am not convinced they are essential to our basic operations."

Bob folded his arms and looked around the table. He hated to be the one to make the hard choices, but thought he was probably the only one in the top level executive group at CareSystems Health Maintenance Organization (HMO) willing to say what needed to be said.

Charlene Bishop, RN, DSN, collected her thoughts. As vice president for patient care, she had 15 MSN-prepared nurses in her division. Seven were certified nurse practitioners who worked with clients in the primary care clinic; three were clinical specialists who operated the community outreach/home health department; and one was a nurse midwife. The remaining four were case managers and managers of the occupational health service, the hospital continuity service, and the quality improvement program. In addition, 30 bachelor of science in nursing–prepared community health nurses worked with the clinical specialists to deliver care.

What was the best way to refute Bob's position, Charlene wondered?

Thoughts & Notes

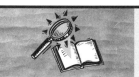 **Case Analysis**
Charlene Bishop

1. What are the concepts covered in the case?

2. What do you know about the case? What actual information do you have?

3. What are your provisional hypotheses?

4. What do you need to know to better understand the concepts or to solve the problem? What are the learning issues?

After answering the above questions for this part of the case, go to Part Two.

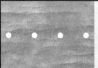

Case Study 4A • Part Two
Charlene Bishop

Case Material

Historically, CareSystems HMO had been a leader in providing innovative, cost-effective health care to the community. It was started in 1975, shortly after the initial passage of federal HMO legislation. The founders were a young activist physician and her best friend, who had served as a community developer with the Peace Corps. CareSystems was the first HMO agency in the state to hire nurse practitioners (NPs) and community health clinical specialists and generalists.

Co-founder Dr. Joyce Smithers felt strongly that a good deal of everyday medical practice could be safely provided by physician extenders. She was happy to hire two diploma-prepared nurses who had attended a 6-month NP certificate program. These nurses were well-accepted by clients, and quickly became integral team members. Problems arose when they attempted to see their clients in the hospital, though, because staff nurses refused to follow their written or verbal orders and hospital administrators would not give them admitting privileges.

In 1976, a certified nurse midwife interviewed at CareSystems. She was relocating to Madisontown and hoped to establish a midwifery service there. Friends had told her that CareSystems was probably the only agency that would consider a midwifery service, and due to its progressive reputation, there was probably a good chance of CareSystems doing so.

To her dismay, Dr. Smithers flatly refused, saying that midwives were unsafe and she had no intention of offering lower quality services at CareSystems. She did finally agree to employ a couple of community health clinical nurse specialists, who she thought would be able to function as nurse practitioners/physician extenders.

Thoughts & Notes

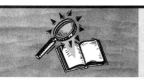

Case Analysis
Charlene Bishop

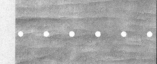

1. What are the concepts covered in the case?

2. What do you know about the case? What actual information do you have?

3. What are your provisional hypotheses?

4. What do you need to know to better understand the concepts or to solve the problem? What are the learning issues?

After answering the above questions for this part of the case, go to Part Three.

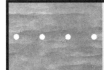 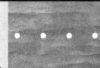

Case Study 4A • Part Three
Charlene Bishop

Case Material

Durand Insurance Co. acquired CareSystems in 1992 during a wave of health care mergers and acquisitions. Durand, a large insurance company, was publicly owned and quite profitable. CareSystems enrollees and employees worried a great deal about the acquisition, fearing that patient care would suffer in a proprietary environment, that employees would lose their jobs, and that clients would lose the benefit of community/home health care and case management.

Many analysts in the Pacific Northwest, where CareSystems was located, were convinced that HMOs were going to be the only way to contain medical costs. Some argued that HMOs would be the foundation of national health insurance. It was not clear at the time whether advanced practice nurses and community health generalists would be utilized more or less at CareSystems.

Thoughts & Notes

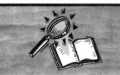

Case Analysis
Charlene Bishop

1. What are the concepts covered in the case?

2. What do you know about the case? What actual information do you have?

3. What are your provisional hypotheses?

4. What do you need to know to better understand the concepts or to solve the problem? What are the learning issues?

After answering the above questions for this part of the case, go to Part Four.

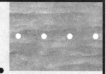

Case Study 4A • Part Four
Charlene Bishop

Case Material

Throughout the 1990s, health administrators began hiring increasing numbers of advanced practice nurses (APNs), believing that expert nurses were cost-effective because of their high levels of productivity compared with other categories of staff. Schools of nursing graduated many different types of nurse practitioners and clinical specialists. CareSystems had finally hired a nurse midwife, although it took a long time to obtain the needed hospital credentialing.

Charlene graduated with a degree as a plastic surgery nurse practitioner and worked for several years with a plastic surgeon. She became dissatisfied with what she saw as a fairly limited role and returned to school to obtain her doctor of science in nursing, majoring in nursing administration.

Charlene joined CareSystems in 1993 in the midst of a budget crisis that had grown worse over time. Primary care physicians were in short supply. Those employed by CareSystems were paid based on the number of clients in their caseloads, so they had little reason to want to share clients with APNs. Charlene worried about quality of care with such an emphasis on numbers and the bottom line.

Now she found herself constantly defending why the HMO's clients needed professional nursing care from BSN-prepared community health nurse generalists as well as care from APNs.

Thoughts & Notes

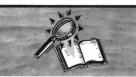 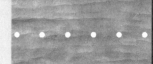

Case Analysis
Charlene Bishop

1. What are the concepts covered in the case?

2. What do you know about the case? What actual information do you have?

3. What are your provisional hypotheses?

4. What do you need to know to better understand the concepts or to solve the problem? What are the learning issues?

After answering the above questions for this part of the case, go to Part Five.

 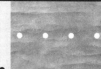

Case Study 4A • Part Five
Charlene Bishop

Case Material

The clientele at CareSystems had changed considerably since the HMO was first formed. Rather than the primarily well-educated, upper-income white clients the HMO had originally attracted, now the client mix was far more diverse.

Janice Applebee, a community health clinical nurse specialist (CNS), had gathered data from the agency's Management Information System (MIS) that showed that 50% of the clients were Caucasian; 20% were African-American (and of those, 5% were Hispanic); another 20% were Hispanic (but not African-American); and 10% of the clients were Aleutian Eskimo. Charlene believed that the diversity represented by the client mix required the skills of community health clinical nurse specialists to balance multiple, potentially conflicting needs, priorities, and optimal interventions.

Janice and one of the nurse managers at CareSystems had shown particular sensitivity to these issues by developing and implementing special outreach programs for minority populations using the community health nurse generalists. Charlene defended the importance of these programs to the chief financial officer, who did not agree that outreach to medically indigent clients was appropriate for an agency that was in severe fiscal crisis.

Thoughts & Notes

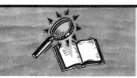 

Case Analysis
Charlene Bishop

1. What are the concepts covered in the case?

2. What do you know about the case? What actual information do you have?

3. What are your provisional hypotheses?

4. What do you need to know to better understand the concepts or to solve the problem? What are the learning issues?

After answering the above questions for this part of the case, go to Part Six.

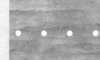

Case Study 4A • Part Six
Charlene Bishop

Conclusion

Meanwhile, at the top level executive group meeting, Charlene leaned forward and said, "As you know, Bob, MSN nurses are one of our most critical assets because they have been shown to be cost-effective and to deliver high quality health care. Community health nurse generalists have been shown to have a positive effect on outcomes of care, such as improved prenatal care and birth outcomes. Here is my plan for reorganization."

Thoughts & Notes

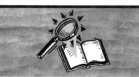 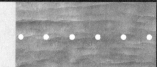

Case Analysis
Charlene Bishop

1. What are the concepts covered in the case?

2. What do you know about the case? What actual information do you have?

3. What are your provisional hypotheses?

4. What do you need to know to better understand the concepts or to solve the problem? What are the learning issues?

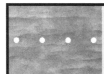

Case Study 4B • Part One
Mary

Mary, a community health nurse generalist, sat in her car recording notes from the home visit she had just made to Mrs. McCoy. "I don't know how much more of this I can take!" she thought. "It just gets harder and harder to give my patients the care that they really need."

Mary thought back to her visit. During the bath, Mrs. McCoy had started crying. "My daughter's husband lost his job last week," she said. "He's taking the whole family up to Metropolis because he heard they were hiring at one of the plants up there. They're talking about putting me in a nursing home because nobody can come out and fix my meals any more. I'd rather die."

Mary sighed. Last month Mr. Wrightwood's family had left, too. They hired a neighbor lady to take care of him, but she didn't have a car. After work, Mary had to run into Center City to buy groceries for him and pick up his prescriptions. Mary sighed again. It was against agency policy to run errands for clients on company time, so she waited until after work. "Let's see," she thought. "That makes seven people I'm doing things for . . ." Mary thought about the team meeting she was late for. "I wonder if the community health clinical nurse specialist can help."

· · · · · *Thoughts & Notes* · · · · ·

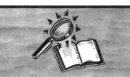 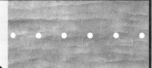

Case Analysis
Mary

1. What are the concepts covered in the case?

2. What do you know about the case? What actual information do you have?

3. What are your provisional hypotheses?

4. What do you need to know to better understand the concepts or to solve the problem? What are the learning issues?

After answering the above questions for this part of the case, go to Part Two.

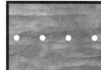 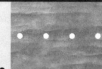

Case Study 4B • Part Two
Mary

Case Material

Lee Harrison, the community health clinical nurse specialist, and Mary were deep in conversation as they walked into the weekly staff meeting of the Casper County Health Department. Lee said, "Why don't you give me some more information about what you're finding in the field to take to the next meeting of the interagency council. We're looking at ways to improve case management in the Medicaid Waiver Program by working with people from housing and social services."

"I thought it was a health council!" exclaimed Mary. "It is," Lee laughed. "But we enlarged our definition of the health care system several years ago. When we decided to try to go to primary health care, we realized we had to work with other sectors of the community, too. Anyway, I know most of your clients are not in the Waiver Program, but I think the council might be in a position to address some of the problems you're describing. I'd like to share your clients' stories with them."

J.J. Crump, the director of nursing, asked, "Do you think they could help with our prenatal patients? I had hoped health care reform would improve access to prenatal care, but now I'm not so sure."

Jon Walters, the family nurse practitioner, turned around and asked, "By the way, is there any truth to the rumor that the nurse midwife setting up practice in Center City is interested in working with underserved populations?"

Lee brightened. "Yes, I talked with her on the phone yesterday. She'll be at the interagency council next week to talk about funding, among other things. Would you like me to invite her to a staff meeting?"

"Oh, yes! Please do!" Mary said. "At our home care team meeting we were talking about the increasing number of referrals that we are getting for high-risk infants. We were wondering what the health department could do to promote better prenatal outcomes. Maybe she could help."

Lee said, "Here comes Dr. Baker to start the staff meeting. Why don't we talk more about this later."

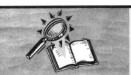 

Case Analysis
Mary

1. What are the concepts covered in the case?

2. What do you know about the case? What actual information do you have?

3. What are your provisional hypotheses?

4. What do you need to know to better understand the concepts or to solve the problem? What are the learning issues?

After answering the above questions for this part of the case, go to Part Three.

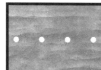

Case Study 4B • Part Three
Mary

Case Material

"The monthly meeting of the Quad-County Interagency Health Services Council will now come to order!" Dr. Baker banged the gavel on the table. "Is there continuing business to be discussed?"

"Yes," said Reba Smith from Jason County Procare. "We were talking about documenting the need for home meal services for people living in rural areas. Our new director of managed care checked with the nursing home in Center City and found that at least 10 of their patients could be on home care if meals were available to them. They all qualify under the Medicaid Waiver Program. What do you think?"

Lee looked around the room at the representatives from the other agencies and thought to herself, "Managed care, hmm. Maybe that's why they're doing so well. If we don't get better funding for the health department, we won't be providing *any* services. I'll have to touch base with Reba later."

Lee turned her attention back to the meeting. Pulling out the notes from her needs assessment of Casper County, she joined in the discussion.

"And now let me introduce our new nurse midwife, Jodie Jackson," Dr. Baker said. "Jodie has just returned from South Africa and is setting up practice in Center City. I think she has some ideas that we might find interesting."

Lee listened carefully as Jodie talked about her proposal for reducing the morbidity and mortality rates in the region.

Thoughts & Notes

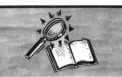 

Case Analysis
Mary

1. What are the concepts covered in the case?

2. What do you know about the case? What actual information do you have?

3. What are your provisional hypotheses?

4. What do you need to know to better understand the concepts or to solve the problem? What are the learning issues?

After answering the above questions for this part of the case, go to Part Four.

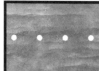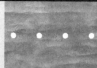

Case Study 4B • Part Four
Mary

Conclusion

There was a knock on the door. "Come in," J.J. called, and Lee, Mary, and Jon entered. "You all look pretty happy," J.J. said.

Mary, Lee and Jon grinned at each other. "We just got back from walking Jodie to her car," Lee said. "She's as excited as we are about what happened in the staff meeting. Dr. Baker was really in favor of Jodie's idea for a regional maternal-child health network. It will help us so much with our own programs."

"Yes," said Mary, "and Lee's report about the Tri-County Interagency Council was really interesting, too. I was excited when she told us about their decision to conduct a regional needs assessment to help plan a regional managed care system. I can't wait. It will have answers to so many of my clients' problems."

"Mmmmm, yes, it will help," said J.J. "But don't forget, change takes time."

Thoughts & Notes

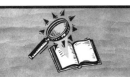 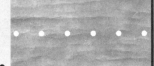

Case Analysis
Mary

1. What are the concepts covered in the case?

2. What do you know about the case? What actual information do you have?

3. What are your provisional hypotheses?

4. What do you need to know to better understand the concepts or to solve the problem? What are the learning issues?

Case Study 4C • Part One
Mrs. Beatty

Case Material

Beth, Dan, Jamie, and Leigh, a new cohort of community health nursing generalists, are involved in an orientation to the local health department.

The four nurses represent a mix of personalities as well as nursing experiences. Beth, an assertive feminist, has a goal of becoming a nurse midwife after working the past 2 years in the Peace Corps in Haiti. Dan really wanted to go to medical school, but after being rejected three times became a nurse and worked on the intensive care unit (ICU) in a tertiary care facility for 5 years. His goal is to become a family nurse practitioner.

Jamie, a quiet, dependable nurse with 12 years of previous experience in a large county health department, is pursuing a goal as a community health nurse clinical specialist. Leigh, who wants to be a director of nursing, comes with a background in clinical and middle management with a visiting nurse association, where her most recent position was assistant director. She is highly motivated and directed in her professional goals toward an administrative role. Her employer urged her to "get an MBA or MHA," but Leigh decided to pursue her education in nursing.

They are all familiar with what the professional literature says about advanced practice roles, and they believe their clinical goals can be achieved through graduate nursing education. They are eager to begin the next two phases of their nursing careers, first as community health nurse generalists and then as graduate students.

Thoughts & Notes

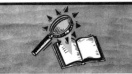

Case Analysis
Mrs. Beatty

1. What are the concepts covered in the case?

2. What do you know about the case? What actual information do you have?

3. What are your provisional hypotheses?

4. What do you need to know to better understand the concepts or to solve the problem? What are the learning issues?

After answering the above questions for this part of the case, go to Part Two.

Case Study 4C • Part Two
Mrs. Beatty

Case Material

Mrs. Beatty arrived at the community clinic with her 3-year-old twins. One was a bit listless; both had poor appetites as compared with their older sibling at the same age. One of the twins complained of stomachaches. The other seemed more irritable, but according to the mother, "that kid always was more high strung than his brother."

Her current pregnancy requires her to rest because of hypertension. As a result, much of the supervision of the twins falls to their 6-year-old sister.

Gwen, the nursing supervisor, presented this information to the four community health nursing generalists. "Now, then," she said, "where would each of you begin? What do you think is going on here?"

· · · · · · *Thoughts & Notes* · · · · ·

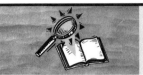

Case Analysis
Mrs. Beatty

1. What are the concepts covered in the case?

2. What do you know about the case? What actual information do you have?

3. What are your provisional hypotheses?

4. What do you need to know to better understand the concepts or to solve the problem? What are the learning issues?

After answering the above questions for this part of the case, go to Part Three.

Case Study 4C • Part Three
Mrs. Beatty

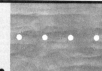

Case Material

Some general discussion followed during which Beth, Dan, Jamie, and Leigh asked questions. Then Gwen added the following information.

Mrs. Beatty's husband works in maintenance for the local university and his health insurance is a basic Blue Cross plan. Mrs. Beatty reports that their apartment is large enough, even for the expected baby, but the landlord does not maintain it well.

"We need a good paint job," she said. "The old stuff is falling off the walls." As to her pregnancy, Mrs. Beatty related that it was unplanned but, "now that it's here, I'm going through with it. No more, though!"

Thoughts & Notes

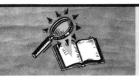 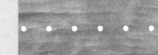

Case Analysis
Mrs. Beatty

1. What are the concepts covered in the case?

2. What do you know about the case? What actual information do you have?

3. What are your provisional hypotheses?

4. What do you need to know to better understand the concepts or to solve the problem? What are the learning issues?

After answering the above questions for this part of the case, go to Part Four.

Case Study 4C • Part Four
Mrs. Beatty

Conclusion

Beth, Dan, Jamie, and Leigh began to discuss the problem the twins presented. "What was the cause?" they asked each other.

Each of the nurse generalists probed the issues around the case from the perspective of his or her own specialty interests. Dan replied first, saying, "I read someplace that family nurse practitioners (FNPs) can prescribe treatment, but we can't do that in this state." Jamie raised questions about the flaking paint problem and asked who should get involved besides the nurse or the health department.

Beth related that while Mrs. Beatty's situation was interesting, her focus would be on this pregnancy. Leigh said that "getting advanced practice nurses (APNs) paid for their services and family planning is important."

· · · · · Thoughts & Notes · · · · ·

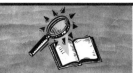 

Case Analysis
Mrs. Beatty

1. What are the concepts covered in the case?

2. What do you know about the case? What actual information do you have?

3. What are your provisional hypotheses?

4. What do you need to know to better understand the concepts or to solve the problem? What are the learning issues?

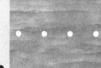

Case Study 4D • Part One
Alice McDermott

Case Material

Alice McDermott, RN, has worked at the Burley County Health Department Clinic for 3 years as a community health nurse generalist. She has noticed that most of her adult clients either have heart disease or die prematurely of cancer. She spends much of her time teaching clients about proper nutrition, smoking cessation, and physical fitness. Although most of her clients express interest and appreciation for her health teaching, few actually change their health habits.

At the annual American Public Health Association (APHA) meeting, Alice meets Karla, a community health clinical specialist who practices at the Burley County Hospital. Karla is concerned about the high incidence of low birthweight (LBW) babies born in Burley County.

· · · · · · *Thoughts & Notes* · · · · ·

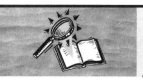 

Case Analysis
Alice McDermott

1. What are the concepts covered in the case?

2. What do you know about the case? What actual information do you have?

3. What are your provisional hypotheses?

4. What do you need to know to better understand the concepts or to solve the problem? What are the learning issues?

After answering the above questions for this part of the case, go to Part Two.

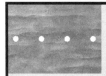 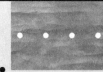

Case Study 4D • Part Two
Alice McDermott

Case Material

Alice and Karla become good friends during the meeting. They are both mothers of school-aged children and are involved in their children's schools. Karla is a member of the parents' council at R.J. Rollin Middle School, where her daughter is a sixth grader. Karla tells Alice that her daughter won't go into the bathroom at school because "it stinks of smoke all the time."

Alice and Karla decide to visit the exhibit area. There are so many new ideas to learn and talk about. They notice a large fluorescent sign about a conference-sponsored "Day at the State Capitol": "Visit the Capitol and have lunch with your legislator. Discuss your concerns with those who make the decisions that affect your practice!"

Thoughts & Notes

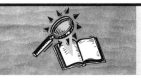

Case Analysis
Alice McDermott

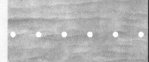

1. What are the concepts covered in the case?

2. What do you know about the case? What actual information do you have?

3. What are your provisional hypotheses?

4. What do you need to know to better understand the concepts or to solve the problem? What are the learning issues?

After answering the above questions for this part of the case, go to Part Three.

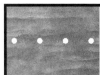 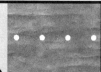

Case Study 4D • Part Three
Alice McDermott

Case Material

Karla and Alice attend a presentation by Jay McKee, RN, MSN, a community clinical nurse specialist; and Pat Treadwell, a master's in public health–trained epidemiologist. Both are from the state Department of Health Services. Jay and Pat compare county mortality data to state and national statistics.

Karla and Alice learn that deaths from heart disease and cancer in Burley County are 3 times the state rate, and that babies born in Burley County are 5 times more likely to be LBW as compared with babies born elsewhere in the state. Karla and Alice are alarmed to learn that 45% of Burley County adults smoke cigarettes, as compared with 27% of state residents. Jay briefly mentions that tobacco farming is the major industry in Burley County.

After a long day of meetings, Karla and Alice pass by a crowded room. Struck by an atmosphere of enthusiasm, they walk in and find nurses learning about how best to influence health policy. Although Alice "hates politics," Karla convinces her to stay.

Thoughts & Notes

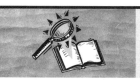 

Case Analysis
Alice McDermott

1. What are the concepts covered in the case?

2. What do you know about the case? What actual information do you have?

3. What are your provisional hypotheses?

4. What do you need to know to better understand the concepts or to solve the problem? What are the learning issues?

After answering the above questions for this part of the case, go to Part Four.

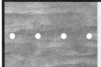 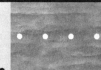

Case Study 4D • Part Four
Alice McDermott

Conclusion

After the public health meeting, Alice and Karla come to the conclusion that smoking is a major problem contributing to heart disease, cancer, and LBW in Burley County. They agree to attack the problem in several different ways. Not only do they incorporate complete tobacco use histories into their direct care routines, but they also evaluate the effectiveness of existing smoking cessation programs in Burley County.

They quickly realize that they cannot effect broad-based change alone. They learn about a group of professionals and citizens who are also concerned about the health effects of tobacco use in Burley County. Alice and Karla join the group and are successful in convincing the county schools to adopt a smoke-free environment policy.

The following year at the APHA meeting, Alice and Karla present the paper: "Finding common ground—How community health nurses can influence health policy."

Thoughts & Notes

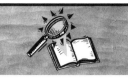

Case Analysis
Alice McDermott

1. What are the concepts covered in the case?

2. What do you know about the case? What actual information do you have?

3. What are your provisional hypotheses?

4. What do you need to know to better understand the concepts or to solve the problem? What are the learning issues?

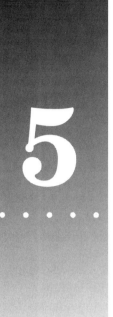

5 Epidemiology in Nursing Practice

Margaret "Peggy" Hickman

Epidemiology is an interdisciplinary science used by health professionals to study the occurrence of health and illness in various populations and settings. The goal of epidemiology is to prevent and control disease and injury. Originally, epidemiology was most closely associated with communicable disease surveillance and control. Current epidemiological methods are used to study and prevent or control the full spectrum of health problems, including acute and chronic communicable and non-communicable diseases and injuries.

Nurses use epidemiological concepts and methods in a variety of practice settings. For example, nurses help prevent communicable diseases of childhood through immunization programs in clinics, preschools, and other community settings. In schools and industrial settings, nurses try to reduce absenteeism through primary and secondary prevention strategies that target individual and group behaviors as well as the environment. In public health settings, nurses are involved in the investigation and control of communicable disease outbreaks.

Nurses also are involved in analyzing and interpreting epidemiological data for clinical use. Infection control nurses are responsible for collecting and analyzing epidemiological data and using their findings to prevent or control nosocomial infections in hospitals and nursing homes. Nurses also participate in planning and evaluating health care services that address the prevailing needs of the community, and take part in evaluating the outcomes of various interventions. In public health and case management settings, nurses use epidemiology to identify populations at risk for illness and injury and to track the outcomes of health promotion and health care programs. Occupational health nurses use epidemiological methods to identify the causes of work-related injuries or illnesses and to develop subsequent occupational injury prevention programs. Finally, nurses are part of surveillance and research teams that monitor health and illness in populations, study the characteristics of acute and chronic health problems, and identify emerging infectious diseases.

This chapter explores epidemiological concepts and methods and the use of epidemiology in nursing practice. The first case focuses on communicable disease control, whereas the second case examines the use of data to plan and evaluate nursing programs. Because epidemiology is a basic public health science, the cases use health departments as the practice setting. However, the skills and knowledge learned in these cases are applicable to a wide variety of health care and community settings. The cases also emphasize the interdisciplinary nature of epidemiology. Nurse generalists and nurse specialists collaborate with each other and with other health professionals in local and state health agencies.

Case Study 5A, Newport Outbreak, provides an overview of how nurses in a health department setting might apply epidemiological concepts and methods to investigate and control an infectious disease outbreak. The setting is a small rural community. Key characters include two public health nurses and a public health physician, all of whom work in a county health department. When a significant number of community members develop gastrointestinal symptoms, the public health team begins the process of investigation and control. Epidemiological methods, including appropriate biostatistical measures, are used to identify the cause of the outbreak and to prevent secondary spread. The case concludes as the team uses appropriate epidemiological language and format to develop a report of their findings and interventions for the board of health.

In Case Study 5B, Urban County, employees (including nurses) of a metropolitan health department use epidemiological data to plan and evaluate health promotion and disease prevention programs for their county. The case explores the types and sources of existing data that can be used to plan and evaluate nursing and other health care services. The methods of using data to analyze health care trends and to forecast their impact on future health services utilization are also implicit in the case. The case can be used to understand the roles and responsibilities of both team leadership and team membership in health care planning. Because of the epidemiological approach, and its reliance on existing data, this case does not include the full range of knowledge and skills needed for health planning. However, it does illustrate the basic epidemiological foundation for comprehensive community health promotion activities, including health assessment and planning, that is found in subsequent chapters.

Resources

Written Resources:

- Epidemiology and biostatistics texts
- State/provincial and local health departments
- State/provincial and county morbidity and mortality data
- State/provincial and county vital statistics
- State and national Behavioral Risk Factor Surveillance System data
- State/provincial and national health objectives

People Resources:

- State commissioner of health
- State nurse epidemiologist
- Local health department nurses
- Staff in vital statistics offices of local and state/provincial health departments

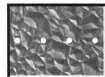 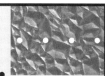

Case Study 5A • Part One
Newport Outbreak

Case Material

Maggie Jones, BSN, pushed her chair back from her desk, stretched, and glanced at the calendar. "October 7. It's been a year and a half since I moved here from the city. Time sure flies when you enjoy what you're doing." She looked at the clock. "The afternoon's more than half gone already. I'd better get back to this paperwork, or I'll never get out of here on time."

As Maggie turned back to her desk, the phone rang. "Hayes County Health Department, Maggie Jones speaking. Yes. Yes. All of you are sick? Yes, I will. Do you feel well enough to give me a little more information?" Maggie frowned as the other phone started ringing. Just then, Rusty Wilson, BSN, came around the corner. Maggie pointed at the ringing phone and mouthed, "Would you get that?"

At 5:00 PM Maggie and Rusty finally put their phones down. "It looks like we have an epidemic on our hands," Maggie said. "Do you think there's anyone over in Newport Corners who hasn't developed acute nausea, vomiting, and diarrhea this afternoon?"

Rusty was counting the names on the phone report. "Well, we have calls from all 24 residents, but believe it or not, only 12 of them are actually sick. A while ago it seemed like everyone in the county was calling us. Maybe we'd better call this an outbreak."

Maggie reached for the public health nursing manual. "I need to brush up on the guidelines for an epidemiological investigation," she said. "I know we covered this in my senior community health nursing (CHN) course 2 years ago. But this is my first chance to participate in an investigation. Do you want me to read aloud?"

Thoughts & Notes

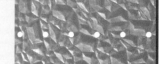

Case Analysis
Newport Outbreak

1. What are the concepts covered in the case?

2. What do you know about the case? What actual information do you have?

3. What are your provisional hypotheses?

4. What do you need to know to better understand the concepts or to solve the problem? What are the learning issues?

After answering the above questions for this part of the case, go to Part Two.

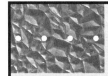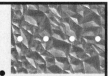

Case Study 5A • Part Two
Newport Outbreak

Case Material

Maggie and Rusty walked toward the parking lot. "Are you sure we have everything we'll need?" asked Maggie.

Rusty frowned in concentration. "I think so," he said. "I double-checked with the state and the Centers for Disease Control and Prevention. We will do the interviews, so I have divided up the names. Dr. Naisbitt is ready to order the recommended lab tests, and I have the containers. The state lab is ready for the onslaught. I think we're all set."

"Let's get going then," said Maggie. "Altogether we have 24 people who attended community meal activities during the past several weeks. What are the dates again?"

Rusty checked his notes. "There was the Founder's Day Picnic at the park on October 4; the potluck supper at the church on October 5; the banquet at the restaurant on October 6; and the Civic Leadership Breakfast at the school on October 7."

Thoughts & Notes

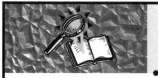 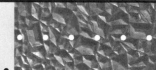

Case Analysis
Newport Outbreak

1. What are the concepts covered in the case?

2. What do you know about the case? What actual information do you have?

3. What are your provisional hypotheses?

4. What do you need to better understand the concepts or to know to solve the problem? What are the learning issues?

After answering the above questions for this part of the case, go to Part Three.

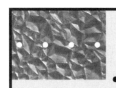 **Case Study 5A • Part Three**
Newport Outbreak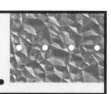

TABLE 5A-1   Summary of Interviews: Characteristics, Onset, and Intake of People Attending Community Meal Functions

Case No./ Description	Symptom Onset	Picnic	Potluck	Banquet	Breakfast
1. 18-year-old male	Oct. 7 at 3 PM	hamburgers, chips, slaw, cake, cola	meatloaf, corn, coffee, mashed potatoes, pie	chicken ala king, peas, green salad, sherbet	eggs, bacon, roll, fresh fruit, coffee
2. 27-year-old female	Oct. 7 at 3 PM	hot dogs, chips, slaw, cake, cola	chicken, green beans, tea, mashed potatoes, pie	chicken ala king, peas, green salad, sherbet	pancakes, sausage, juice, roll, coffee
3. 18-year-old female	none	hamburgers, chips, slaw, cake, cola	meatloaf, corn, water, mashed potatoes, pie	chicken ala king, peas, green salad, sherbet	eggs, bacon, roll, fresh fruit, coffee
4. 29-year-old male	none	hot dogs, chips, slaw, cake, cola	chicken, corn, coffee, mashed potatoes, pie	pot roast, peas, green salad, sherbet	pancakes, sausage, juice, roll, coffee
5. 31-year-old male	Oct. 7 at 3 PM	hamburgers, chips, slaw, cake, cola	meatloaf, beans, tea, mashed potatoes, pie	chicken ala king, peas, green salad, sherbet	eggs, bacon, roll, fresh fruit, coffee
6. 33-year-old female	Oct. 7 at 3 PM	hot dogs, chips, slaw, cake, cola	chicken, corn, water, mashed potatoes, pie	chicken ala king, peas, green salad, sherbet	pancakes, sausage, juice, roll, coffee
7. 37-year-old male	none	hamburgers, chips, slaw, cake, cola	meatloaf, corn, coffee, mashed potatoes, pie	pot roast, peas, green salad, sherbet	eggs, bacon, roll, fresh fruit, coffee
8. 31-year-old female	none	hot dogs, chips, slaw, cake, cola	chicken, green beans, tea, mashed potatoes, pie	chicken ala king, peas, green salad, sherbet	pancakes, sausage, juice, roll, coffee
9. 37-year-old male	Oct. 7 at 3 PM	hamburgers, chips, slaw, cake, cola	meatloaf, corn, water, mashed potatoes, pie	pot roast, potatoes, green salad, sherbet	eggs, bacon, roll, fresh fruit, coffee
10. 41-year-old female	Oct. 7 at 3 PM	hot dogs, chips, slaw, cake, cola	chicken, corn, coffee, mashed potatoes, pie	chicken ala king, peas, green salad, sherbet	pancakes, sausage, juice, roll, coffee
11. 42-year-old female	none	hamburgers, chips, slaw, cake, cola	meatloaf, beans, tea, mashed potatoes, pie	pot roast, peas, green salad, sherbet	eggs, bacon, roll, fresh fruit, coffee
12. 45-year-old male	none	hot dogs, chips, slaw, cake, cola	chicken, green beans, tea, mashed potatoes, pie	pot roast, peas, green salad, sherbet	pancakes, sausage, juice, roll, coffee

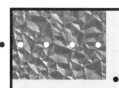 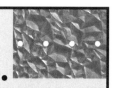

Case Study 5A • Part Three
Newport Outbreak—cont'd

13. 46-year-old female	Oct. 7 at 3 PM	hamburgers, chips, slaw, cake, cola	meatloaf, corn, coffee, mashed potatoes, pie	chicken ala king, peas, green salad, sherbet	eggs, bacon, roll, fresh fruit, coffee
14. 47-year-old male	Oct. 7 at 3 PM	hot dogs, chips, slaw, cake, cola	chicken, corn, water, mashed potatoes, pie	chicken ala king, peas, green salad, sherbet	pancakes, sausage, juice, roll, coffee
15. 42-year-old female	none	hamburgers, chips, slaw, cake, cola	meatloaf, beans, tea, mashed potatoes, pie	pot roast, peas, green salad, sherbet	eggs, bacon, roll, fresh fruit, coffee
16. 45-year-old male	none	hot dogs, chips, slaw, cake, cola	chicken, corn, coffee, mashed potatoes, pie	pot roast, peas, green salad, sherbet	pancakes, sausage, juice, roll, coffee
17. 58-year-old female	Oct. 7 at 3 PM	hamburgers, chips, slaw, cake, cola	meatloaf, corn, water, mashed potatoes, pie	chicken ala king, peas, green salad, sherbet	eggs, bacon, roll, fresh fruit, coffee
18. 59-year-old female	Oct. 7 at 3 PM	hot dogs, chips, slaw, cake, cola	chicken, green beans, tea, mashed potatoes, pie	chicken ala king, peas, green salad, sherbet	pancakes, sausage, juice, roll, coffee
19. 58-year-old male	none	hamburgers, chips, slaw, cake, cola	meatloaf, corn, coffee, mashed potatoes, pie	pot roast, peas, green salad, sherbet	eggs, bacon, roll, fresh fruit, coffee
20. 59-year-old female	none	hot dogs, chips, slaw, cake, cola	chicken, green beans, tea, mashed potatoes, pie	pot roast, peas, green salad, sherbet	pancakes, sausage, juice, roll, coffee
21. 68-year-old female	Oct. 7 at 3 PM	hamburgers, chips, slaw, cake, cola	meatloaf, corn, water, mashed potatoes, pie	chicken ala king, peas, green salad, sherbet	eggs, bacon, roll, fresh fruit, coffee
22. 72-year-old female	Oct. 7 at 3 PM	hot dogs, chips, slaw, cake, cola	chicken, green beans, tea, mashed potatoes, pie	chicken ala king, peas, green salad, sherbet	pancakes, sausage, juice, roll, coffee
23. 65-year-old female	none	hamburgers, chips, slaw, cake, cola	meatloaf, corn, water, mashed potatoes, pie	pot roast, peas, green salad, sherbet	eggs, bacon, roll, fresh fruit, coffee
24. 79-year-old male	none	hot dogs, chips, slaw, cake, cola	chicken, corn, coffee, mashed potatoes, pie	pot roast, peas, green salad, sherbet	pancakes, sausage, juice, roll, coffee

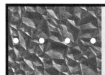 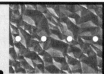

Case Study 5A • Part Four
Newport Outbreak

Case Material

Maggie and Rusty shuffled the case interview reports back and forth across the table. "The individual reports don't tell me anything more than the summary table," said Rusty. "What do you think of that epidemic curve we just calculated?"

"I think it's the strangest looking epidemic curve I've ever seen," replied Maggie. "Dr. Naisbitt, what do you think about this?"

"I think you'd better back to work on those attack rates and frequency tables," said Dr. Naisbitt. "I need to get a profile of person, place, and time, as well as aggregates at risk."

"I know, I know," Maggie said. "But really—what do you think caused the outbreak?"

"Well, I won't rule anything out for now, but we might want to look at some of the usual suspects," the doctor said. "What do you think of this lineup: *Staphyloccus aureus, Clostridium perfringens,* gastroenteral virus, *Salmonella,* and *Shigella?*"

"I think you were right when you said we'd better get back to work," said Maggie. "I'd like to recheck the attack rates for each food item. After all, the agent is only a part of the picture.

"I guess what I'm really asking is why do you think all those people got sick? Newport Corners has a lot of community activities that involve meals, but we've never had an outbreak like this before. I thought the county had a pretty good primary prevention system in place. I wonder what happened."

Thoughts & Notes

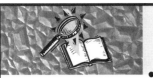 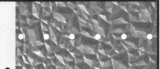

Case Analysis
Newport Outbreak

1. What are the concepts covered in the case?

2. What do you know about the case? What actual information do you have?

3. What are your provisional hypotheses?

4. What do you need to know to better understand the concepts or to solve the problem? What are the learning issues?

After answering the above questions for this part of the case, go to Part Five.

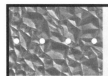 **Case Study 5A • Part Five**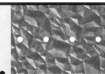
Newport Outbreak

Conclusion

Maggie, Rusty, and Dr. Naisbitt sat around the table in the lunch room. Maggie and Rusty looked at the lab reports and smiled at each other. "Just as we suspected, *Salmonella!* Are we good detectives or what?" Maggie said.

"You mean good public health nurses," Dr. Naisbitt said. "I'm glad you two were able to use your epidemiological skills to help the team control this outbreak so effectively. Without the fast action in putting the secondary prevention measures into place, it could have been a lot worse."

Maggie and Rusty grinned. "Thanks, Dr. Naisbitt. Just doing our job," Rusty said.

"And speaking of our job," Dr. Naisbitt continued, "there's still some unfinished . . ."

"Paperwork!" Maggie and Rusty groaned in unison.

"I'm afraid so," smiled Dr. Naisbitt. "The county board of health meets in 2 weeks, and they want to know what caused the outbreak, who was at risk, and what you did. I want you to be there to give the report.

"Bring a brief, typed report of your investigation. You can attach any charts, graphs, or tables that you think would make the report clearer. I think the board would be interested in your preliminary hypothesis and how you tested it.

"I'm proud of you two," the doctor said. "I know the board hired you with home health care in mind. But I think your report will give a clear picture of how public health nurses can benefit the county by focusing on prevention at the aggregate level."

Thoughts & Notes

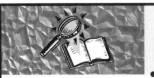 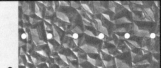

Case Analysis
Newport Outbreak

1. What are the concepts covered in the case?

2. What do you know about the case? What actual information do you have?

3. What are your provisional hypotheses?

4. What do you need to know to better understand the concepts or to solve the problem? What are the learning issues?

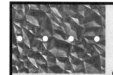 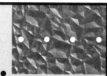

Case Study 5B • Part One
Urban County

Case Material

Brenda and Joe looked at each other across their piles of records. "What do you think about our new assignment?" Joe asked.

Brenda shook her head and smiled. "I don't know," she said. "I've been hoping that the health department would hire a nurse specialist to work with us. I guess I hadn't realized I'd be asking to do more paperwork. Why can't we find out the county's health needs by looking at our caseloads?"

The phone rang. "Urban County Health Department. Public Health Nursing," Joe said, then listened for a minute. "Just a minute and I'll ask," he said. "Brenda, Ronnie is getting ready for our working meeting and wants to know if we have any questions. Do you have any?"

"I don't think so," she said. "We're supposed to look at the various sources of epidemiological data for the county and decide what can best help us identify the county's major health problems. Right?"

"Right," he said, turning back to the phone. "Nope, no questions. We'll see you later at the staff meeting."

• • • • • • *Thoughts & Notes* • • • • •

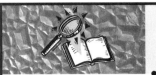
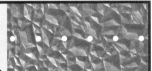

Case Analysis
Urban County

1. What are the concepts covered in the case?

2. What do you know about the case? What actual information do you have?

3. What are your provisional hypotheses?

4. What do you need to know to better understand the concepts or to solve the problem? What are the learning issues?

After answering the above questions for this part of the case, go to Part Two.

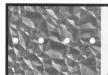 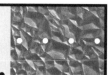

Case Study 5B • Part Two
Urban County

Case Material

"Well, what do you think?" Ronnie asked.

Joe looked doubtfully at the papers he and Brenda had been passing back and forth. "I'm not sure what I'm supposed to be thinking about," he said. "We have demographic data, morbidity data, mortality data, and vital statistics. I'm feeling a bit overwhelmed."

"Sorry," Ronnie laughed. "I've been pulling together these data a little bit at a time. I forgot how overwhelming it looks when you see it all at once. Let's back up for a minute.

"Start with the latest mortality data," he said. "First, let's look at the leading causes of death for the county as a whole. Got that page? Now, I'd like you to think about several things. First of all, what are the major health problems that people in Urban County are dying from?"

He paused while they studied this information, then continued. "Why don't you both make notes of this. We'll be using this information a little later. Now look at our rates compared with the state as a whole. What do you think?"

Again he waited while they pondered the data. "OK, now let's break it down the same way by age group. What do you think?" He paused. "Brenda, why are you frowning?"

"Well, this stuff is interesting," she said, "but I'm working in maternal and child health (MCH). I'd been hoping to see something that fits more with what I'm doing. Are MCH data available too?"

Thoughts & Notes

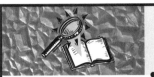 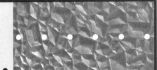

Case Analysis
Urban County

1. What are the concepts covered in the case?

2. What do you know about the case? What actual information do you have?

3. What are your provisional hypotheses?

4. What do you need to know to better understand the concepts or to solve the problem? What are the learning issues?

After answering the above questions for this part of the case, go to Part Three.

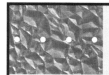 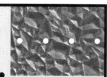

Case Study 5B • Part Three
Urban County

Case Material

"Joe, what do you think about these rates?" Ronnie asked.

"They are starting to make sense to me," he said. "Did you see how Urban County compares with some of the more rural counties in our health district?"

"Yes," Ronnie said, "I've been looking at Farmer and Mountain counties. The differences are interesting. What do you think, Brenda?"

"I'm amazed at our own county," she said. "My caseload has been mostly MCH and communicable diseases. I guess I've been a bit narrow in my view of what we need to be doing as nurses. I haven't changed my mind about the importance of MCH and communicable disease control; but based on these rates, I think we need to be doing more to prevent chronic diseases."

"Actually, that's one of the reasons I wanted to meet with you," Ronnie said. "Dr. Gramrock says the health department needs to address the national goals of increasing the span of healthy life and reducing health disparities. He and the director of nursing are working on the new 5-year plan with these goals in mind.

"They are looking at Urban County in relation to the state and national health objectives for both health promotion and preventive services. They would like our input about what we think the priorities for nursing services should be."

Thoughts & Notes

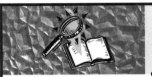 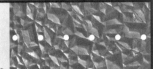

Case Analysis
Urban County

1. What are the concepts covered in the case?

2. What do you know about the case? What actual information do you have?

3. What are your provisional hypotheses?

4. What do you need to know to better understand the concepts or to solve the problem? What are the learning issues?

After answering the above questions for this part of the case, go to Part Four.

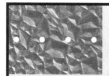 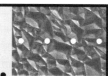

Case Study 5B • Part Four
Urban County

Case Material

Ronnie looked at Joe and Brenda. "I want to make sure we are in agreement," he said. "We have agreed to expand our priorities to include heart disease, cancer, and cerebrovascular disease prevention. Is that correct?"

"Yes," Brenda said, "but we decided to keep MCH promotion services, too."

Ronnie smiled at her. "That's right," he said. "Now, based on the trends, are there any other health problems we should be considering?"

"Given predicted changes in Urban County's demography and economic base, I think we should consider some of the health problems related to 'dys-ease,'" Brenda said. "That is the discomfort some persons have in accepting certain illnesses like acquired immunodeficiency syndrome (AIDS)."

Joe added, "I don't think we can forget the communicable diseases either. The trends for AIDS and tuberculosis are scary."

"All right, we'll add them to the list." Ronnie said. "Now, let's talk about the nursing services needed for primary prevention of these health problems. Have you had a chance to look at some of the risk factors yet?"

Joe said, "The summaries from the health risk appraisals we've been doing in our clinics and outreach sites aren't available yet, but we've been looking at the state's behavioral risk factor survey for our area. I think it has some useful information."

Thoughts & Notes

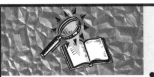 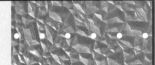

Case Analysis
Urban County

1. What are the concepts covered in the case?

2. What do you know about the case? What actual information do you have?

3. What are your provisional hypotheses?

4. What do you need to know to better understand the concepts or to solve the problem? What are the learning issues?

After answering the above questions for this part of the case, go to Part Five.

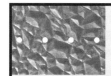 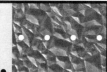

Case Study 5B • Part Five
Urban County

Conclusion

Ronnie straightened the books and papers into a neat pile. "This is a good beginning," he said. "We've used the county's epidemiological data to identify some of the major trends and health problems. I think we have an idea of what is endemic to Urban County. Let's begin to map out some strategies for nursing care.

"Given the range of nursing services, I think we should address prevention at the individual and family levels, as well as at the community level. Do you want to use an ecological model or an environmental model to put our ideas together?"

Thoughts & Notes

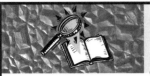 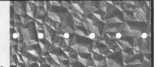

Case Analysis
Urban County

1. What are the concepts covered in the case?

2. What do you know about the case? What actual information do you have?

3. What are your provisional hypotheses?

4. What do you need to know to better understand the concepts or to solve the problem? What are the learning issues?

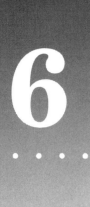

6 Family and Community Health Promotion

Marilyn Givens King

Today's nurse faces a rapidly changing health care delivery system. Themes that characterize these changes include (1) shorter hospital stays, (2) a movement toward community-based health care delivery, (3) managed health care systems, (4) a shifting emphasis from illness to wellness, and (5) greater reliance on families to provide a significant portion of nursing and health care services. While these changes offer tremendous opportunities to influence the types and quality of health care services available to communities, there is a concomitant need for the nurse to acquire a different set of skills than those traditionally required by the in-patient setting. In addition to the traditional knowledge about pathophysiology, pharmacology, and nursing care of ill individuals, nurses also require a solid grounding in family and community theories, as well as theories of health promotion and disease prevention. Family and community assessment strategies, critical analysis of assessment data bases to identify assets and needs, and expertise in working with families and community groups are important additions to the nurse's lexicon of practice skills.

The case studies in this chapter address (1) family assessment and issues family caregivers face in providing care for their loved ones, (2) community health assessment and strategies for working with population groups, and (3) family health promotion within a community setting.

Case Study 6A, The Goldmark Family, is about a family in the "sandwich generation" dealing with the declining health and increasing dependency of an aging parent as well as the demands of growing children. This is a complex case that involves many issues related to individuals and families as they affect the health of a given family. It explores important nursing content relating to working with families, nursing assessment of families, identification of health status indicators, and community resources.

Case Study 6B, Juel County, examines a variety of concepts, frameworks, and methods that can be used in the process of designing and implementing a comprehensive and collaborative community health assessment at the state or county level. In this case, a community health clinical nurse specialist has been asked to conduct an assessment of a rural county to determine unmet health needs and the impact of a possible structural/organizational change. Theories and conceptual models are explored for use as potential frameworks for practice.

The final case study in this unit, Dee's Dilemma, focuses broadly on family and community health promotion and builds on the concepts covered in the previous cases. In this complex situation, a community health nurse applies health promotion concepts within the context of a multi-problem family. Whereas the case initially directs attention to the Martinez family, the nurse eventually realizes that other families in the migrant community are dealing with similar problems and expands her work to the community level. Through work with informal community leaders, peer support groups are developed as a method of providing health promotion education.

In summary, the case studies in this unit are designed to provide the student with a conceptual and theoretical basis in the practice of family and community health nursing with a specific focus on assessment and health promotion strategies.

Resources

Electronic Resources: Web sites

Census Bureau	http://www.census.gov
Centers for Disease Control	http://www.cdc.gov
World Health Organization (WHO)	http://www.who.org
Healthy Cities USA	http://www.who.org/peh/ccs/CCsData/ amro/USA/Indianapolis.htm
Healthy Cities WHO	http://www.who.dk/tech/hcp/index.htm

People Resources:

1. Interview nurses in your community who work with families. Find out how they assess families, what types of family problems they most often encounter, and how they intervene to promote family health. Home health agencies, public health departments, occupational health services, or adult day care are examples of community settings where such nurses might be employed.
2. Interview a nurse working at a state or provincial health department about health policies that support family functioning and family well-being.
3. Identify and interview a family currently caring for an elderly family member with a chronic health problem. Ask the family what it is like caring for this family member. How has this experience changed their lives? What strategies and what community resources have the family used to cope?
4. Obtain community assessment information from the local chamber of commerce, health department, or area development district (or other local economic development office). Compare the information obtained from different agencies with your own observations obtained through a windshield survey.

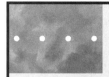 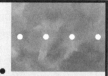

Case Study 6A • Part One
The Goldmark Family

Case Material

"My mother-in-law just can't stay by herself any longer" Janet Goldmark told Joe Yost, RN, a community health nurse generalist.

"She isn't safe alone. But Dan—my husband—doesn't see it. He thinks if we just hire someone to stay with her during the day, she will be OK. I'm afraid that she will either fall or leave the stove on and start a fire.

"On the other hand, I don't know what else we can do. Dan and his sister, Martha, definitely wouldn't consider putting their mother in a nursing home. And if we bring her to our house, I don't know what I will do. I have my hands full with my job and taking care of Sara and Ashley. You know, a couple of preschool age children can be a handful." Janet looked extremely anxious and her eyes began to fill with tears.

Joe began to review the family history on the chart. After he skimmed the pages, he looked up at Janet. "Can you tell me a little more about your family?" he asked.

Goldmark Family History

Nuclear Family: Dan Goldmark, 45 years; Janet Goldmark, 40 years; their children Ashley, 4 years, and Sara, 2 years

Extended Family: Ruth, Dan's mother, 75 years; Martha, Dan's sister, 48 years

Recent social history: Dan lost his job 1 month ago. The local area is economically depressed and the prospects for a new job at the same salary are not good.

Janet began working at a local department store 1 year ago. Initially, she just worked 2 days a week, but has been working almost full time since Dan was laid off. She hopes to obtain a regular full time position soon so she can become eligible for benefits.

The family attends church about once a month. They do not have many close friends at the church.

The family lives in a 3-bedroom house in a middle-income neighborhood. The house has 1100 square feet of living space.

Usual Interaction Patterns: Dan is the usual decision maker about financial issues. Janet defers to him, although she occasionally seems irritated by having to do so.

Janet is responsible for all child care and decisions regarding the children. Dan seems puzzled at times by her insistence that he help make some of the child-rearing decisions.

Janet and Dan are good friends with one couple who live in their neighborhood. They also visit some old college friends about once each year in a city an hour and a half away.

Health history: Dan was diagnosed with hypertension 2 years ago. He is taking medication for it.

Janet is in good health, except for chronic headaches which she has been told are stress-related.

Both children are in good health. Sara has frequent ear infections and Ashley seems to have developed allergies, although the family does not yet know what she is allergic to. They hope to have her tested soon.

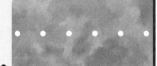

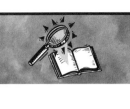

Case Analysis
The Goldmark Family

1. What are the concepts covered in the case?

2. What do you know about the case? What actual information do you have?

3. What are your provisional hypotheses?

4. What do you need to know to better understand the concepts or to solve the problem? What are the learning issues?

After answering the above questions for this part of the case, go to Part Two.

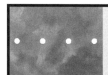 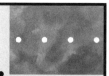

Case Study 6A • Part Two
The Goldmark Family

Case Material

"Dan was laid off from his job at the bank last month," Janet sobbed. "He had a good job—he was a senior account analyst—so we have some money saved. But things look bad for bankers right now, and I just don't know how long our savings will last.

"We are really depending on my job, and that just puts so much pressure on me. Especially now, with Dan's mother not doing well. It seems like everyone is depending on me. I don't know how well we can all hold up under this kind of stress."

"Is there anyone you can ask for help?" inquired Joe.

"No, not really" Janet said. "Dan's sister, Martha, is the only other family member, and she lives so far away. Besides, Martha and her mother don't get along. Martha is gay and lives with her partner, and her mother really disapproves.

"If we only had to worry about Dan's job, we might be able to manage. But now, thinking about taking care of his mother at our house really means I will do most of the caregiving. I just wish I knew what to do."

· · · · · Thoughts & Notes · · · · ·

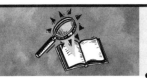

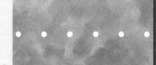

Case Analysis
The Goldmark Family

1. What are the concepts covered in the case?

2. What do you know about the case? What actual information do you have?

3. What are your provisional hypotheses?

4. What do you need to know to better understand the concepts or to solve the problem? What are the learning issues?

After answering the above questions for this part of the case, go to Part Three.

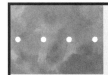 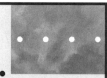

Case Study 6A • Part Three
The Goldmark Family

Case Material

One month later, Joe saw Janet and Dan Goldmark at the clinic. They had brought Ruth, Dan's mother, in to get a flu shot and to have her evaluated because she was getting increasingly forgetful. During his assessment of the family, Joe learned that Janet and Dan had decided to bring Ruth to stay with them for a few weeks so they could find out more about her health status and determine whether she could continue to live in her own home.

Ruth did not completely understand the reason for her stay with her son and daughter-in-law, although she enjoyed the opportunity to be with her grandchildren. Since she lived two states away, she did not get to see them as often as she liked.

The visit was not going well. Janet was already exhausted from caring for Ruth. Four-year-old Ashley had moved into 2-year-old Sara's room so Ruth could have a bedroom of her own. Ashley and Sara had been arguing over toys and were both cranky and difficult for Janet to deal with. Janet had called in sick at work several times because the sitter had been unable to come, and her supervisor was getting annoyed with Janet's absences. Ruth wanted to help with the cooking, but often forgot things like turning the stove off or adding crucial ingredients.

Dan couldn't understand why his wife could not manage. He and Janet had had some heated arguments over the situation. Dan thought they should just close Ruth's house up and let her move in with them. Ruth cried when he suggested it, and Janet told Dan later that she wished she could run away.

Thoughts & Notes

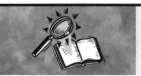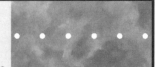

Case Analysis
The Goldmark Family

1. What are the concepts covered in the case?

2. What do you know about the case? What actual information do you have?

3. What are your provisional hypotheses?

4. What do you need to know to better understand the concepts or to solve the problem? What are the learning issues?

After answering the above questions for this part of the case, go to Part Four.

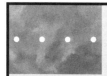
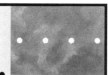

Case Study 6A • Part Four
The Goldmark Family

Case Material

"You know, we have a lot of families like the Goldmarks," Joe remarked to Mike Rowland. Mike was the community health nurse clinical specialist at the Family Care Center, and he and Joe frequently discussed clinical problems. Mike appreciated Joe's creative suggestions for clinical programs, and was happy that Joe initiated development of proposals for new programming.

"We should probably explore what is available in town to help families in the 'sandwich generation,'" Joe said. "If we can't find something to meet our clients' needs, we may want to start something here."

"Why don't you just conduct some classes on caregiving for elderly people?" Mike suggested. "I know of several programs where the nurses teach the families how to do things like bathing and dressing and preparing special diets."

"I don't know," mused Joe. "I think these families need more than classes. I am just not sure what it is, or the best way to help."

Thoughts & Notes

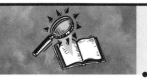 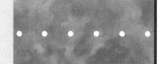

Case Analysis
The Goldmark Family

1. What are the concepts covered in the case?

2. What do you know about the case? What actual information do you have?

3. What are your provisional hypotheses?

4. What do you need to know to better understand the concepts or to solve the problem? What are the learning issues?

After answering the above questions for this part of the case, go to Part Five.

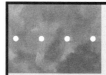
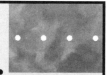

Case Study 6A • Part Five
The Goldmark Family

Conclusion

Six months after Joe's first meeting with Janet Goldmark, he sat down for a family conference with Janet; her husband, Dan; Janet's mother-in-law, Ruth; Dan's sister, Martha (who was visiting); and the two children, Ashley and Sara.

Joe had referred the family to a home care service for assistance with Ruth's personal care needs. They had enrolled Ruth 3 days a week in an adult day-care center where the fee was manageable. Another 2 days a week, a college student stayed with Ruth while Janet was at work.

Dan had gotten a new job with a large banking firm and was pleased with his salary. Martha had agreed to contribute financially to her mother's care, and the family learned that Ruth's savings were adequate to help with some of the caregiving expenses.

The family agreed that things were stable for now, and Ruth indicated that she was content with the situation. Joe and the family concluded that their major emphasis now should be on planning for the future when Ruth's condition might worsen.

Thoughts & Notes

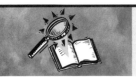

Case Analysis
The Goldmark Family

1. What are the concepts covered in the case?

2. What do you know about the case? What actual information do you have?

3. What are your provisional hypotheses?

4. What do you need to know to better understand the concepts or to solve the problem? What are the learning issues?

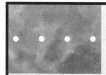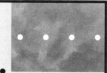

Case Study 6B • Part One
Juel County

Case Material

Dottie Wald, RN, MSN, is a certified community health clinical nurse specialist in independent consulting practice. She has just returned from a meeting with State Health Commissioner Dr. Green, who is concerned about a potential problem with Juel County. Juel County is part of the Essex District Health Department, a 6-county regional health department in a rural part of the state.

The Health Department and the county government have opposing views about the health service needs of the county. The county government has identified some perceived major unmet health needs and has suggested that the Health Department expand its services to provide for these needs. The Health Department responded that it is providing all the services it possibly can within the current budget. The county government then suggested that the Health Department was not using its resources wisely and that Juel County would be better served if it withdrew from the District Health Department and formed an independent unit.

Dr. Green is concerned about the impact of such an action. He asked Dottie to conduct a community assessment and give an objective opinion of the health service needs of Juel County and the desirability of withdrawing from the district. Dottie agreed to do so.

In reviewing her notes from the meeting, Dottie saw that Dr. Green wants her to use the World Health Organization's Outline of Local Health Study (1960) to guide the assessment. She is unfamiliar with the WHO tool, and is also not clear about whether Dr. Green wants an assessment of Juel County or the entire Essex health district. Dottie picks up the phone to call Dr. Green.

Thoughts & Notes

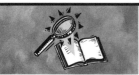 

Case Analysis
Juel County

1. What are the concepts covered in the case?

2. What do you know about the case? What actual information do you have?

3. What are your provisional hypotheses?

4. What do you need to know to better understand the concepts or to solve the problem? What are the learning issues?

After answering the above questions for this part of the case, go to Part Two.

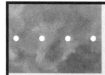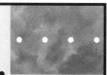

Case Study 6B • Part Two
Juel County

Case Material

Dottie glanced in her rearview mirror as she pulled out of the parking lot of the Juel County Government Complex. She saw Dr. Snow, the county health officer, in animated discussion with Jim Boyd, chairperson of the Health Department Board. With a wry smile, she thought about the meeting she just had with them. . . .

"Hello, I'm Dottie Wald," Dottie had said as she shook hands with the men. "I'm here to discuss an assessment of the health service needs of the county."

Dr. Snow stood up and glared at Dottie. "Who sent you here? Dr. Green?" he demanded. "Well, yes, but . . ." Dottie began. Mr. Boyd chimed in. "Who does he think he is? Does he have jurisdiction over our health department? The state is always telling us what to do!"

Dottie took a deep breath and started over. "I'm a nurse consultant hired by the state to conduct an independent community health assessment of Juel County," she said. "I could do an assessment based on health statistics, but that would only give part of the picture. Most counties have a pretty good idea of what their health needs and resources are. I'd like to include the Juel County perspective in my assessment, and that's why I asked to meet with you. Furthermore, I'm hoping that the information from the assessment will be useful to the county as well as the state."

Dr. Snow sat back down. "You mean you'd tell the state what we think?" he asked. Dottie nodded. "Well, in that case," he said, looking at Mr. Boyd. "What do you think, Jim? Shall we talk to her about this?"

Thoughts & Notes

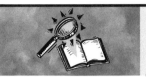

Case Analysis
Juel County

1. What are the concepts covered in the case?

2. What do you know about the case? What actual information do you have?

3. What are your provisional hypotheses?

4. What do you need to know to better understand the concepts or to solve the problem? What are the learning issues?

After answering the above questions for this part of the case, go to Part Three.

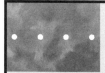 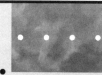

Case Study 6B • Part Three
Juel County

Case Material

Dottie stretched and looked at the calendar. "Two months since we started the assessment," she thought. The door opened and Dottie stood up. "Hello, Dr. Snow, Mr. Boyd," she said. This is a great computer your office complex has. Margie and I just finished setting up your data base."

Margie, the community health nurse generalist with Juel County, planned to have all the assessment data entered in the next week.

"You are fortunate to have a staff member with the assessment and computer skills that Margie has," Dottie smiled. "Margie, why don't you share your questions with Dr. Snow and Mr. Boyd?"

"Well, my main question is, has the committee decided which way it's going to go for planning?" Margie asked.

"When we set up the data base, we made sure that we could input the assessment reports in several different ways. Dr. Green wanted the World Health Organization format. Dr. Snow, I think you wanted to use APEXPH (Assessment Protocol for Excellence in Public Health); and Mr. Boyd, you like PATCH (Planned Approach to Community Health). I'm not sure what the community wanted. They seemed sort of confused about what you wanted to do next."

Three pairs of eyes turned to look at Dottie. She laughed and raised her hands. "Hey, this is your decision, remember? What format would be most helpful to the planning committee?"

Mr. Boyd cleared his throat. "We sort of hoped you would tell us," he said. "After all, you're writing an assessment report, too."

Dottie smiled. "I'm putting my independent assessment in a format that can be used for a variety of planning frameworks," she said. "Tell you what . . . The committee is waiting in the conference room. As soon as Dr. Green gets here, let's talk about the pros and cons of each framework. Then you can decide what best fits Juel County."

Thoughts & Notes

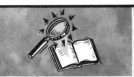 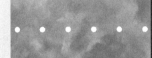

Case Analysis
Juel County

1. What are the concepts covered in the case?

2. What do you know about the case? What actual information do you have?

3. What are your provisional hypotheses?

4. What do you need to know to better understand the concepts or to solve the problem? What are the learning issues?

After answering the above questions for this part of the case, go to Part Four.

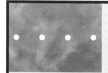 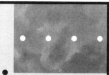

Case Study 6B • Part Four
Juel County

Conclusion

Dottie leaned back in her chair and let the completed report fall onto her desk. "Four months, Margie," she said. "It is hard to believe that so much time has passed since we started working with Juel County.

"I never thought we would see the day when Juel County, the District Health Department, and the state would agree on anything," Dottie said. "But once they decided to compromise and modify APEXPH with WHO components for the assessment, and use the PATCH process for planning, things went more smoothly."

Dottie picked up the report again. "Unmet health needs of Juel County identified by community residents include . . . ." she read. "I guess everybody learned something. I don't know who was more surprised by the community input, Dr. Green or Dr. Snow. I'm glad they finally decided to use a community development approach to health promotion and disease prevention."

Just then the phone rang. "Health Promotion Consultants Incorporated, Dottie Wald speaking."

"Hello, Dottie! This is Dr. Green," the voice on the other end said. "Do I have an opportunity for you! Do you have a minute to talk?"

· · · · · · Thoughts & Notes · · · · ·

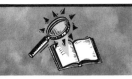

Case Analysis
Juel County

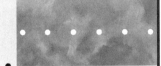

1. What are the concepts covered in the case?

2. What do you know about the case? What actual information do you have?

3. What are your provisional hypotheses?

4. What do you need to know to better understand the concepts or to solve the problem? What are the learning issues?

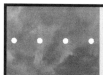 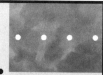

Case Study 6C • Part One
Dee's Dilemma

Case Material

Dee poured a second cup of coffee while Barbara read through Josie Martinez's chart. Both women were relatively new community health nurses at the Pine Creek Community Health Center.

"This is such a difficult situation," Barbara said. "I don't know what you can do right now to make a difference."

Dee nodded. "I have seen Josie twice in the clinic, and she just seems to have given up. How can I help her if she isn't motivated?" she said.

"And she has so many strikes against her," Dee said. "Hector is hardly ever at home, and with five children, Josie is just exhausted. Here she is, pregnant again, 44 years old, and addicted to alcohol. Not only that, but Miguel has been drinking heavily also, and he is only 13. Angie ran away last year and was gone for a week. Can you imagine? She was only 11 at the time.

"Josie acts like it is nothing unusual," Dee said. "What is worse is that there are so many families like this over in the migrant camp.

"I know Mrs. Donnemeyer, the nurse manager, wants us to focus on health promotion with our clients. But that seems unrealistic with these families," said Dee. "The Martinez family has so many problems. Where do we start?"

· · · · · Thoughts & Notes · · · · ·

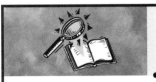 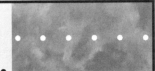

Case Analysis
Dee's Dilemma

1. What are the concepts covered in the case?

2. What do you know about the case? What actual information do you have?

3. What are your provisional hypotheses?

4. What do you need to know to better understand the concepts or to solve the problem? What are the learning issues?

After answering the above questions for this part of the case, go to Part Two.

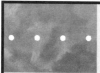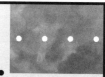

Case Study 6C • Part Two
Dee's Dilemma

Case Material

"Josie, is there any way you can get your three youngest children into the clinic for their shots?" Dee asked. "It's really important for them to complete their immunizations."

As she sat across from Mrs. Martinez in the examination room, Dee wondered if it was fair to discuss immunizations when Mrs. Martinez had so much going on.

"Si, I will do what I can," sighed Josie Martinez. She held her youngest child, 2-year-old José, on her lap. "Is there any way you can help me get stamps for food?" she asked.

"My friend told me I could get stamps, and then maybe the kids could eat a little better," Josie said. "Hector says it's no good to get charity, but I want the kids to have more meat and healthy food. I never have any money, and what I do get from Hector, I have to use—you know?" Mrs. Martinez seemed to be looking to Dee for understanding.

Josie went on. "I talked with the counselor about the drinking, like you said. I don't see how it will do any good, but I'm worried about my baby. I'm afraid the state will take it away if they know I'm drinking when the baby is born."

Thoughts & Notes

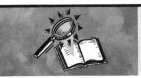 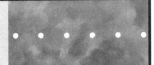

Case Analysis
Dee's Dilemma

1. What are the concepts covered in the case?

2. What do you know about the case? What actual information do you have?

3. What are your provisional hypotheses?

4. What do you need to know to better understand the concepts or to solve the problem? What are the learning issues?

After answering the above questions for this part of the case, go to Part Three.

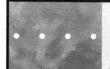
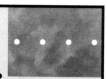

Case Study 6C • Part Three
Dee's Dilemma

Case Material

Two months later, Dee and Barbara were discussing their concerns about health promotion with Mrs. Donnemeyer, the community health nurse manager.

"Mrs. Donnemeyer, some of these families just have so many needs we hardly know where to begin," Dee said. "We know you want us to emphasize health promotion, but that seems like a concept that is foreign to these multiproblem families. In fact, I would say it might be more appropriate if we worked in a setting where we saw more middle-class families who didn't have so many problems."

Marge Donnemeyer took a deep breath. "Perhaps you are being too hasty," she said. "Let's try to think about the needs that some of the families in the migrant camp have in common. Then maybe we can develop a program for many of the families and really make a difference in terms of that community.

"For example, what types of health teaching are you both doing with the families now?"

····· *Thoughts & Notes* ·····

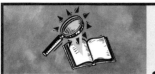

Case Analysis
Dee's Dilemma

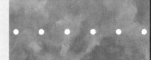

1. What are the concepts covered in the case?

2. What do you know about the case? What actual information do you have?

3. What are your provisional hypotheses?

4. What do you need to know to better understand the concepts or to solve the problem? What are the learning issues?

After answering the above questions for this part of the case, go to Part Four.

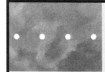
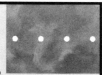

Case Study 6C • Part Four
Dee's Dilemma

Case Material

Dee, Barbara, and Mrs. Donnemeyer eventually developed a peer support program for the families in the migrant camp. Because so many of the families were Hispanic, they enlisted the aid of a lay community health worker who was fluent in Spanish.

At first, the peer support program focused mostly on sharing problems. Gradually, as a few group members began to experience some success with various health promotion activities, they were able to begin functioning as group leaders.

Dee thought the Community Health Center needed to apply for grant funding to expand the program, and she approached Mrs. Donnemeyer about it.

"I think we really need to begin providing training for the group leaders to help them develop their leadership skills so they can mobilize the families in the migrant camp to make decisions about their health," said Dee.

Although Mrs. Donnemeyer was enthusiastic about the grant, she had one concern. "Since most of the families are only in the area for about 4 months at a time, how can we plan for continuity and expect long-lasting effects?" she wondered.

Thoughts & Notes

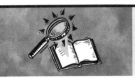 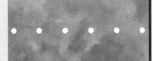

Case Analysis
Dee's Dilemma

1. What are the concepts covered in the case?

2. What do you know about the case? What actual information do you have?

3. What are your provisional hypotheses?

4. What do you need to know to better understand the concepts or to solve the problem? What are the learning issues?

After answering the above questions for this part of the case, go to Part Five.

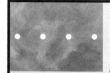 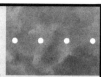

Case Study 6C • Part Five
Dee's Dilemma

Conclusion

Dee and the other nurses at the Pine Creek Community Center submitted a grant to the Public Health Service to expand the peer support program. They used the PATCH model and involved informal leaders in the migrant camp in the decisions about what types of strategies to propose.

Dee was particularly pleased that Josie Martinez volunteered to be a group leader a year after she had her baby. Josie was still being seen by a counselor at the Center for her alcoholism, and acknowledged that she would always have to deal with her disease one day at a time. She had been sober for over a year and had all of her children living with her. Hector had moved on to another migrant camp, and Josie expected to catch up with him in a few months.

Dee thought, "This family is making real progress. The key was convincing Josie to seek alcoholism treatment and empowering her as an active member of the peer support program."

• • • • • Thoughts & Notes • • • • •

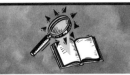

Case Analysis
Dee's Dilemma

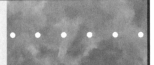

1. What are the concepts covered in the case?

2. What do you know about the case? What actual information do you have?

3. What are your provisional hypotheses?

4. What do you need to know to better understand the concepts or to solve the problem? What are the learning issues?

7 Population-Focused Practice

Margaret "Peggy" Hickman

One of the distinctive characteristics of community health nursing practice is its focus on populations rather than on individuals and families. Health is affected by a variety of factors, such as genetic makeup; social, physical, economic, political, and cultural environment; access to health care; and individual and family behaviors. Population-focused care seeks to improve the health status of communities, states, regions, and the entire nation by addressing the conditions that promote and support wellness and modifying the risks underlying illness.

Health care of populations takes a variety of forms. Community health education aims to increase the knowledge and skills needed to promote and protect health. Issues of improving the environment and access to health care may be addressed by case management, health planning, community development, and health policy. The goal of this chapter is to build the skills and knowledge needed to develop, implement, and evaluate population-focused health promotion interventions. It includes opportunities to analyze the relationships between public health and public health/community health nursing and to examine determinants of public health policy and their impacts on population-focused practice.

The three cases in this chapter address population-based needs assessment, community health planning, and program and policy evaluation.

Case Study 7A, Patty Adams and Her Students, builds on the material in Chapter 6: Family and Community Health Promotion. In this case, a community health nursing faculty member and her students collaborate with members of a low-income community to assess health needs and resources. Public health issues and policies are addressed. The community includes a variety of aggregates that reflect the demographic structure and health risks that must be considered when planning population-focused programs of primary and secondary prevention. Access to health care and the structure of the health care system are also included in the assessment. Finally, it explores how community health nurse specialists and generalists work together in population-focused needs assessment.

Case Study 7B, Parish or Perish, draws upon concepts and methods related to planning population-focused health promotion programs and policies. The case opens as a parish nurse and members of an agricultural community sit down to prioritize community needs and begin the planning process. Community organization and coalition building are introduced as the planning group expands to include other sectors of the community. A variety of programmatic and policy issues are incorporated into the case.

The emphasis of Case Study 7C, Earlene Isom, is on evaluating health policies and programs. Various models and methods are addressed as an occupational health nurse evaluates a worksite-based case management program. Issues such as outcomes, cost-benefit, cost-efficiency, and cost-effectiveness are explored. Public policies related to the case are included as the nurse considers the context in which occupational health programs are developed and implemented. Finally, information management is discussed within the context of health care planning and evaluation.

Collectively, the three cases cover the various stages of population-focused community assessment, community-based health planning, program implementation and evaluation, and policy analysis. The cases also allow an in-depth analysis of how nurse generalists and nurse specialists collaborate with each other, with other professionals, and with members of the community to achieve community-based health goals.

Resources

Written Resources:

- Census data
- State crime data
- State and local morbidity/mortality data
- State worker's compensation data
- State health objectives

People Resources: Persons to interview to clarify case concepts

- Occupational health nurses working in local industry
- Parish/congregational nurses working in local parish communities
- Public health nurses working in local/state health departments
- Sanitarians and environmental specialists
- Health educators
- Safety specialists at state Farm Bureau
- Safety specialists at state Cooperative Extension Service

Electronic Resources:

1. Check state or provincial home pages on the World Wide Web for local data and community/public health planning information.
2. Web sites

Healthy People 2000	http://odphp.osophs.dhhs.gov/pubs/hp2000/
Health Care Financing Administration Statistics	http://www.hcfa.gov/stats/hstats96/ blustcov.htm
Community-Campus Partnerships for Health	http://futurehealth.ucsf.edu/ccph.html

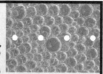

Case Study 7A • Part One
Patty Adams and Her Students

Case Material

Patty Adams, PhD, a community health clinical nurse specialist, sat down with her students for their clinical conference. "We have been asked by Dr. Irene Juneau, the service-learning coordinator, to carry out a community assessment of the public housing project in town to support a grant proposal she is writing," Patty said.

"Our task today is to determine what we already know and how to go about obtaining the needed data. Sharon, you have spent some time at the community center at The Village. What are your observations so far?"

"It is a housing project of 150 two-bedroom townhouse apartments," Sharon said. "The units are small, but appear to be well-maintained. When I drove through the community, I noticed a number of young women visiting while they watched their small children at the playground. I also noticed a few elderly people sitting out on their porches. There were no men about during the times I have been there.

"The first day I was at the community center, I met 2 young women who came in with their children. Laticia, who has 2 small children, told me that she had a miscarriage 2 weeks ago. Toni, a 15-year-old, came into the center with her 1-year-old son. She is 7½ months pregnant with her second baby.

"Toni told me she just had her first prenatal visit 2 weeks ago. She and Laticia both quit school with their first pregnancies and have not returned. I later asked Mrs. Riggs, the director of the center, how these young women support themselves. She told me they each receive Aid to Families with Dependent Children (AFDC) support payments and Medicaid for the children. Toni is also in the Women, Infants, and Children (WIC) program."

Thoughts & Notes

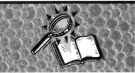 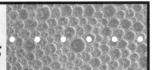

Case Analysis
Patty Adams and Her Students

1. What are the concepts covered in the case?

2. What do you know about the case? What actual information do you have?

3. What are your provisional hypotheses?

4. What do you need to know to better understand the concepts or to solve the problem? What are the learning issues?

After answering the above questions for this part of the case, go to Part Two.

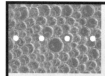 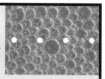

Case Study 7A • Part Two
Patty Adams and Her Students

Case Material

Carla had also spent some time at the community center. Patty asked what she had noticed about sanitation, garbage, and other environmental hazards.

"My first impression was that the apartments are very close together and that there is limited outdoor space," Carla responded.

"I also noticed that there are two large dumpsters located in the center of the complex between two buildings. On the days that I visited, the dumpsters were full and overflowing onto the ground around them. I don't recall paying attention to any smells from that area as I drove by. I also noticed a lot of litter around some of the apartments. I didn't see any rats, but there were some roaches in the kitchen of the community center.

"While I was at the center last week, I spent some time talking with two elderly sisters who live at The Village," Carla continued. "Becky, the oldest, is a retired elementary school teacher. She has problems with hypertension and congestive heart failure. Mary, a retired LPN/LVN, has non–insulin-dependent diabetes mellitus. Later, Ms. Jones, the social worker for the community center, told me that Becky and Mary were both unmarried and that their small pensions were inadequate to meet their living expenses. Becky is 65 and is now on Medicare, but Mary is only 59 and has no health insurance.

"I asked Ms. Jones about the educational and income levels of the residents in general. She said that Mary and Becky were unusual in that they both had post–high school educations. Many of the younger residents have dropped out of school and are on welfare."

Brad asked if she had noticed any evidence of illicit drug problems in the community.

"When I was leaving, I noticed a group of young men hanging out near the playground," Carla said. "It looked like they were passing things back and forth. I felt very uncomfortable and not quite safe observing them."

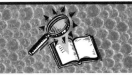 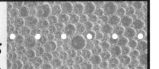

Case Analysis
Patty Adams and Her Students

1. What are the concepts covered in the case?

2. What do you know about the case? What actual information do you have?

3. What are your provisional hypotheses?

4. What do you need to know to better understand the concepts or to solve the problem? What are the learning issues?

After answering the above questions for this part of the case, go to Part Three.

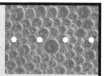

Case Study 7A • Part Three
Patty Adams and Her Students

Case Material

At their next clinical meeting, the students shared the information they had gathered during the intervening week. The quality and amount of data indicated that they had been busy learning how to obtain census data to describe the community. They had also developed a survey questionnaire to gather data from the residents about perceived health problems and sources of health care.

Patty asked all the students to turn their attention to the health care system in the community. "What resources are available to these citizens?" she asked Tena.

"I think that many of the young women go to the health department for their prenatal care and well baby care," Tena said. "There is also a WIC clinic where they can get nutrition supplementation." "There is also the Free Clinic located about a mile from The Village, as well as the outpatient clinics at the hospital," Barbara chimed in.

Patty asked the class about private practitioners in the area. After a moment of silence, Iolene responded, "I'm not real sure about doctors in private practice. Will they see poor people?"

Thoughts & Notes

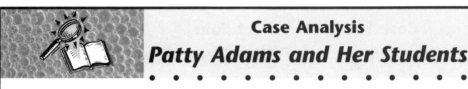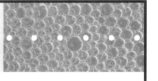

Case Analysis
Patty Adams and Her Students

1. What are the concepts covered in the case?

2. What do you know about the case? What actual information do you have?

3. What are your provisional hypotheses?

4. What do you need to know to better understand the concepts or to solve the problem? What are the learning issues?

After answering the above questions for this part of the case, go to Part Four.

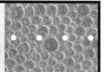

Case Study 7A • Part Four

Patty Adams and Her Students

Conclusion

Patty Adams and her students continued to work on the project. At the end of the semester they turned in a completed report to Dr. Juneau, who was very pleased with the depth and thoroughness of their work.

Their assessment identified a number of needs, such as health promotion activities for the young mothers and their children, that could be addressed by the presence of a nursing clinic on the grounds of the community.

Sharon became quite enthusiastic about the project and community health nursing. At the final conference for the semester she asked, "If I were working as a community health nurse and wanted to develop a health promotion project for this community, what would I do next?"

"That is a very good question," Patty responded. "That is what we will be dealing with next semester."

Thoughts & Notes

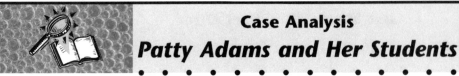

Case Analysis

Patty Adams and Her Students

1. What are the concepts covered in the case?

2. What do you know about the case? What actual information do you have?

3. What are your provisional hypotheses?

4. What do you need to know to better understand the concepts or to solve the problem? What are the learning issues?

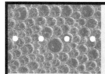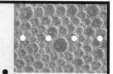

Case Study 7B • Part One
Parish or Perish

Case Material

Leslie Ray, MSN, RN, looked around the advisory group of the Parish Nurse Program. "It's hard to believe that we started the Parish Nurse Program here at Centreville Church 2 years ago," she said. "I brought the summary of our activities that you requested at our last monthly meeting.

"As you can see, our wellness program is well attended during the winter," Leslie said. "People really like the blood pressure screening and Fit After Fifty programs. It's interesting that very few participate during the warm weather months."

"That's because we're all busy on the farm," said Jed Stone, Advisory Committee chairperson. "Maybe we should cancel the wellness program during the summer. After all, farming is a healthy way of life."

Judy Stone tugged on her husband's sleeve. "Depends on whether or not you think getting hurt is healthy," she said. "Just look at how many families the nurse volunteers visited because somebody got hurt on the farm. Last month alone we visited four different families. One of them was a child who got hurt while he was helping with chores after school."

Evelyn Hayes, wife of the county extension agent, nodded. "You're right," she said. "I think almost every family in the church has at least one person who has been injured or killed on the farm. Leslie, isn't there anything you can do?"

Thoughts & Notes

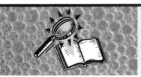 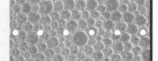

Case Analysis
Parish or Perish

1. What are the concepts covered in the case?

2. What do you know about the case? What actual information do you have?

3. What are your provisional hypotheses?

4. What do you need to know to better understand the concepts or to solve the problem? What are the learning issues?

After answering the above questions for this part of the case, go to Part Two.

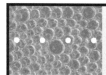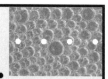

Case Study 7B • Part Two
Parish or Perish

Case Material

"I called the health department last week, but they didn't have any exact figures on farm injuries," Leslie said. "Most of you farm. What have you heard?"

"People get hurt by the equipment, falling off wagons, and getting crushed by their tractors," said Jed. "Tractor rollovers, that's the biggest problem."

Evelyn added, "John, my husband, is always talking to groups about tractor safety. He's a county extension agent, you know. In fact he's giving a talk at the Future Farmers of America (FFA) meeting tonight."

"That's where our grandson is tonight," Jed said. "Now I suppose he'll have something new to nag me about. Last week the Vocational Agricultural teacher told him to wear ear plugs around loud machines. As if they're any louder than his radio."

When the laughter died down, Leslie said, "Sounds like we're not the only ones concerned about farm health. Do you want to work with others in the county on farm health issues, or should we focus our energies on what the church can do?"

The Advisory Committee discussed the issue late into the evening. Finally Jed said, "If we all agree that a community farm safety coalition is the way to go, let's go home."

Thoughts & Notes

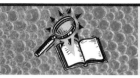 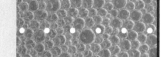

Case Analysis
Parish or Perish

1. What are the concepts covered in the case?

2. What do you know about the case? What actual information do you have?

3. What are your provisional hypotheses?

4. What do you need to know to better understand the concepts or to solve the problem? What are the learning issues?

After answering the above questions for this part of the case, go to Part Three.

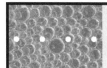 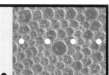

Case Study 7B • Part Three
Parish or Perish

Case Material

Several weeks later, Leslie walked out of the Farm Bureau building with John and Jed. "You two really had some good ideas tonight," she said. "The committee made a good choice in sending you as our representatives to the new Centreville Healthy Farm Family Coalition. What did you think about tonight's meeting?"

"I'm impressed with the injury prevention program that's coming together," Jed answered. "I never thought I'd see the day when we all could agree on any issue in this county."

"It didn't look like we were going to agree about anything for awhile," John laughed. "Didn't I hear someone hollering 'No legislator is going to tell me that I have to use a seat belt on my tractor,' and 'What do you mean I can't carry the grandkids in my lap when I plow?' That was a pretty good speech."

Jed, embarrassed, said, "Guess I got carried away. But I think most of us would rather do these things because we want to, not because the government says we have to. I really liked the idea about seeing if the health insurance companies will give a price break to Healthy Farm Family Coalition members who participate in our safety program."

• • • • • • *Thoughts & Notes* • • • • • •

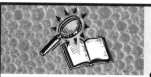 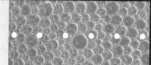

Case Analysis
Parish or Perish

1. What are the concepts covered in the case?

2. What do you know about the case? What actual information do you have?

3. What are your provisional hypotheses?

4. What do you need to know to better understand the concepts or to solve the problem? What are the learning issues?

After answering the above questions for this part of the case, go to Part Four.

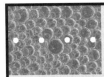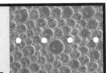

Case Study 7B • Part Four
Parish or Perish

Conclusion

Jed called the monthly meeting of the Parish Nursing Advisory Committee to order. "Let's go ahead and begin," he said. "We have a full agenda."

He talked about the Farm Bureau's policy role in supporting farm health and safety promotion as part of a state health plan. When he finished, John described the joint educational program being started by the Cooperative Extension Service, the schools, and the county health department.

Evelyn nodded. "I took John's farm safety videos for the health department to show in the waiting room when I took Kelsey in for her shots last week. They were really glad to get them."

Leslie listened to the enthusiasm of the committee and thought, "A lot of people are really involved in the Coalition's farm health and safety activities. But I wonder if we are really making a difference."

• • • • • • Thoughts & Notes • • • • • •

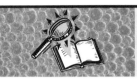

Case Analysis
Parish or Perish

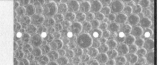

1. What are the concepts covered in the case?

2. What do you know about the case? What actual information do you have?

3. What are your provisional hypotheses?

4. What do you need to know to better understand the concepts or to solve the problem? What are the learning issues?

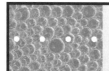 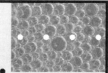

Case Study 7C • Part One
Earlene Isom

Case Material

Earlene Isom is a master's-prepared occupational health nurse working for a mining company located in Keating County, a county of 3000 people. Earlene began a case management program for adults receiving Workers' Compensation for black lung disease 1 year ago. Many of her clients also have tuberculosis (TB). After seeing how quickly her caseload grew over the first 6 months, she became concerned about the need to decrease the overall incidence and prevalence of black lung disease and TB.

Earlene persuaded the mining company to underwrite the cost of a prevention program aimed at workers, who were not always following the company's safety policies; and at supervisors, who sometimes cut corners with safety requirements. This program also focused on TB prevention in the community as a company-sponsored community service. She named the program Clean Air, Clean Lungs.

The company has strongly supported the Workers' Compensation case management program because Earlene has been able to demonstrate how much money it is saving in Workers' Compensation costs. However, Don Elam, the company manager, told her last week that money was getting tight because of the decreasing market for coal, and that he might not be able to fund the Clean Air, Clean Lungs program next year. Earlene had been thinking that she needed to evaluate this program in a more formal way, and now she knew it was essential. Earlene scheduled a meeting with her staff nurse, Tena, to begin work on this.

Thoughts & Notes

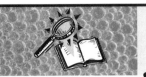 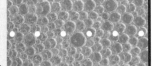

Case Analysis
Earlene Isom

1. What are the concepts covered in the case?

2. What do you know about the case? What actual information do you have?

3. What are your provisional hypotheses?

4. What do you need to know to better understand the concepts or to solve the problem? What are the learning issues?

After answering the above questions for this part of the case, go to Part Two.

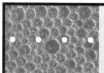 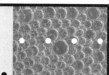

Case Study 7C • Part Two
Earlene Isom

Case Material

Earlene decided to begin her program evaluation by looking at the goals and objectives of the Clean Air, Clean Lungs program. The program goals were to:

1. Reduce company costs for coal worker's pneumoconiosis (CWP).
2. Reduce the incidence of CWP among company employees.
3. Reduce the incidence of TB in Keating County.
4. Develop standards to prevent CWP among company employees.

The program objectives were to:

1. Increase the percentage of company managers who comply with safety policies related to coal dust by 50% within 2 years.
2. Increase the percentage of employees who follow safety rules related to coal dust by 50% within 2 years.
3. Decrease the costs associated with Workers' Compensation claims for CWP.
4. Conduct community screenings for TB in Keating County.

Earlene asked Tena to begin putting together a list of the activities related to the program's objectives

Thoughts & Notes

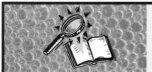 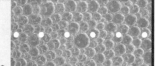

Case Analysis
Earlene Isom

1. What are the concepts covered in the case?

2. What do you know about the case? What actual information do you have?

3. What are your provisional hypotheses?

4. What do you need to know to better understand the concepts or to solve the problem? What are the learning issues?

After answering the above questions for this part of the case, go to Part Three.

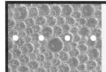 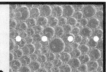

Case Study 7C • Part Three
Earlene Isom

Conclusion

One week after beginning to plan the evaluation of the Clean Air, Clean Lungs program, Earlene became concerned that she would not be able to demonstrate that the program effectively reduced company expenses.

She thought the program was a good one, and that people both in the community and at the mine were learning more about all three levels of prevention in relation to CWP and TB. However, she worried that her objective to reduce company expenses may have been too optimistic. Also, Earlene thought that the employees may be at higher risk for developing both CWP and TB in part because their lungs were already damaged by smoking. Finally, she talked with the human immunodeficiency virus (HIV) program coordinator at the health department and learned that the number of people in the county who were HIV-positive was increasing.

One of Earlene's biggest concerns was how to collect and manage the data she needed for evaluating this program. She knew a bit about using spreadsheets for data management and had once prepared a data codebook for a research class; but other than that, she was not sure where to begin.

Thoughts & Notes

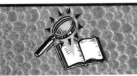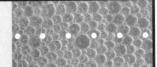

Case Analysis
Earlene Isom

1. What are the concepts covered in the case?

2. What do you know about the case? What actual information do you have?

3. What are your provisional hypotheses?

4. What do you need to know to better understand the concepts or to solve the problem? What are the learning issues?

Issues in Rural Nursing

Marilyn Givens King

"Why do I need to know about rural people and rural health? I don't plan to live and work in a rural area," the student nurse from a large urban area might say. Or, the student who grew up on a farm might ask, "Why do I need to study about rural health problems and issues? I've always lived in a rural area. I know these people and what the life there is like." On the surface these seem like reasonable questions. After all, aren't rural people just like people everywhere? The only difference is that there are fewer people in rural areas and, hence, fewer things to do!

The reality is that there are some important differences between rural and urban environments that influence an individual or family's access to health care and that may affect the desired outcomes of care. These differences include culture, geography, limited health care resources, state and national health care policies, and transportation. An appreciation and understanding of these issues will provide nurses with the skills needed to provide culturally sensitive quality nursing care to all people.

The case studies in this chapter are designed to address these issues. Case Study 8A, Janice Bryan Moves to the Mountains, is about a nurse who moves with her husband from a large city to a rural community. This complex case provides an opportunity for students to explore a variety of issues in rural nursing. On one level, Janice Bryan is struggling with the confusion of trying to live and work in a culture she does not understand. At the same time, the health problems she faces provide an opportunity to investigate the role of the public health nurse in providing care to individuals, families, and the community.

Case Study 8B, Rural Home Health Care, is the story of a nurse confronted with the conflict between the needs of a family and the limitations of their health insurance coverage. The nurse, Connie, is faced with an all-too-common scenario when she visits George Barnett, who has end-stage Alzheimer's disease, and finds his daughter at her wits' end. Connie's challenge is to find the resources to help this family cope with the demands of a debilitating illness.

In summary, this chapter provides an overview of the many issues that impact the delivery of quality health care to rural populations. Whether the care is delivered in an urban tertiary care hospital or a small rural home health agency, an understanding of the rural health, social, economic, and cultural environment will enhance the quality of services rendered.

Resources

Electronic Resources: Web sites

National Rural Health Association   http://www.nrharural.org
Rural Health Network   http://www.uchsc.edu/sm/sm/
    rural/index.htm

National Center for Health Statistics   http://www.cdc.gov/
    nchswww/default.htm

People Resources:

1. Interview a home health administrator about reimbursement policies and the impact of changes in these policies on the ability to provide services to patients and families.
2. Interview a few health providers about their ability to coordinate services for their clients. What are the issues involved in the coordination of care in a rural community? What is the role of case management in rural health settings?
3. Identify and interview informal community leaders about the culture of their community and how this affects the delivery of and access to health care services.

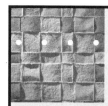
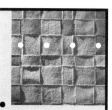

Case Study 8A • Part One
Janice Bryan Moves to the Mountains

Case Material

Janice Bryan, BSN, RN, was born and raised in New York City. She has worked as a public health nurse since her graduation from nursing school. Now 28 years old, she has been married for 2 years. Her husband, Jimmy Johnson, grew up in the mountains but moved to New York when he was laid off from his job with the coal mines. Jimmy was not satisfied living away from his family and the hills. He secured a job with a solid waste disposal company planning to establish a landfill near his home, and he and Janice moved back. Janice was offered and accepted a job at the local health department.

During her orientation, Carol Cunningham, MSN, RN, explained to Janice that the region is very rural and mountainous, with limited health care services and resources available. There are many barriers to the delivery of health care, including the geography, isolation, poverty, and the culture of the region.

"What do you know about rural culture and mores?" Carol asked.

Janice answered, "I know very little. I've always lived in a large city and went to school there. I don't recall my professors talking with us about rural issues."

Carol replied, "Then I can see you will need some orientation to this."

Two weeks later, Janice was talking with Carol about some problems she was having. "The other nurses here aren't very helpful. Every time I ask them to help me with something, they all say, 'Sure, I don't care to.' I don't understand why they don't want to be helpful."

Carol chuckled, then explained. "You have just encountered the colloquial use of language. In this area that phrase means 'I'll be happy to help you.' Sit down and let's discuss this further. Have you encountered any other phrases or words that seem to mean something different from what you think it means?"

Thoughts & Notes

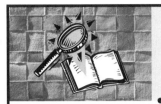

Case Analysis
Janice Bryan Moves to the Mountains

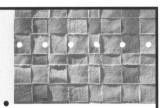

1. What are the concepts covered in the case?

2. What do you know about the case? What actual information do you have?

3. What are your provisional hypotheses?

4. What do you need to know to better understand the concepts or to solve the problem? What are the learning issues?

After answering the above questions for this part of the case, go to Part Two.

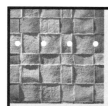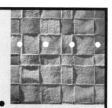

Case Study 8A • Part Two
Janice Bryan Moves to the Mountains

Case Material

After 1 month on the job, Janice approached Carol. "Do you have a few minutes to talk?" she said. "I've just come back from visiting the Arnett family and need some help to understand what I'm seeing and how to help them."

"Sure," Carol replied. "Tell me what's going on with the Arnetts."

"I made a visit to follow up with Mrs. Arnett about her positive TB skin test," Janice began. "It was a terrible drive out there. They live 2 miles up a one-lane dirt road that is also used by trucks hauling coal from a strip mine near the Arnett's home. At times I couldn't see the road for the dust, and it was washed out in several places from recent flooding.

"When I finally got to their house, I noticed several beat-up cars in the yard, only one of which worked, Mrs. Arnett said. I also noticed several discarded appliances sitting in the yard. When I got out of the car, the air smelled of sewage. The ditch in front of the house was full of water, but I couldn't tell where it was coming from.

"The inside of the house was fairly clean, although there were pop cans, bags of chips, and cookies left out. They have no hot water, and use kerosene heaters to heat the house. Several of these were placed around the house. I guess I was shocked to see that people live in this kind of environment.

"I have worked with poor people before, but this is just different. In New York, the residents of housing projects often have to put up with roaches, inadequate plumbing, and other such problems. But they don't own their apartments and have little control over their landlords. Here, the Arnett family owns their home and property, but just doesn't seem to care."

"Let's see if we can help you gain some perspective on what you are seeing here," Carol replied. "What do you think are the economic and social realities for this family?"

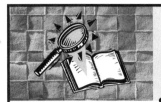 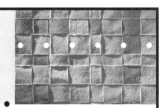

Case Analysis
Janice Bryan Moves to the Mountains

1. What are the concepts covered in the case?

2. What do you know about the case? What actual information do you have?

3. What are your provisional hypotheses?

4. What do you need to know to better understand the concepts or to solve the problem? What are the learning issues?

After answering the above questions for this part of the case, go to Part Three.

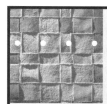

Case Study 8A • Part Three
Janice Bryan Moves to the Mountains

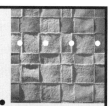

Case Material

"I'm feeling frustrated in trying to help this family," Janice continued. "They don't follow my advice. I had told Mrs. Arnett that all of her family needed to get a purified protein derivative (PPD) test, but none of the family came in to be tested. When I asked about this, Mrs. Arnett said that her son didn't see a need for testing because the rest of the family felt fine. She also said her son was afraid the test might cause them to get TB. Later, Mrs. Arnett told me she had quit taking her medication because it made her sick.

"Mrs. A's 17-year-old granddaughter, Sharon, came in, so I had a chance to talk with her," Janice said. "I learned that Sharon is a single mother with a 2-year-old daughter whose name is Tammy. She said she has never taken Tammy in for immunizations because she can't afford a regular doctor and doesn't trust the health department. She uses her grandmother's old-time remedies when Tammy gets sick."

"It sounds like there are a lot of health issues going on with the Arnett family that need to be addressed," Carol said. "I think this family would make a good case study for our staff meeting next week. Maybe we can come up with a plan and strategies to help you work with the Arnetts."

The following week Janice presented her case at the weekly staff meeting. Several of the other nurses shared similar experiences. "What suggestions do you have for Janice to help her work with the Arnett family?" Carol asked.

Thoughts & Notes

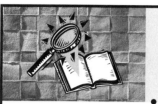

Case Analysis
Janice Bryan Moves to the Mountains

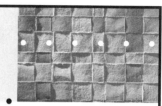

1. What are the concepts covered in the case?

2. What do you know about the case? What actual information do you have?

3. What are your provisional hypotheses?

4. What do you need to know to better understand the concepts or to solve the problem? What are the learning issues?

After answering the above questions for this part of the case, go to Part Four.

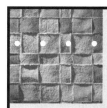 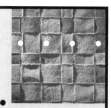

Case Study 8A • Part Four
Janice Bryan Moves to the Mountains

Case Material

The staff had a lengthy discussion about possible approaches Janice could use with the Arnetts. Then Mary Jamison, RN, MSN, the director of nursing, said, "I'm very concerned about how these cases of TB are going to affect our community.

"The number of cases has tripled in the last year. We are seeing more cases where people aren't responding to the usual medications. We are seeing more immigrants moving into this area, and we also have a large population of elderly people residing here.

"The living conditions of many of these people only make treatment more complicated. I think we need to spend some time talking about the needs of the larger community and how we begin to address this problem. It's important to be concerned about individual families, but there is a bigger community problem arising here."

Picking up on Mary's comments, Carol asked, "What do you think our next steps should be?"

Thoughts & Notes

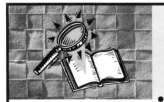
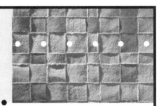

Case Analysis
Janice Bryan Moves to the Mountains

1. What are the concepts covered in the case?

2. What do you know about the case? What actual information do you have?

3. What are your provisional hypotheses?

4. What do you need to know to better understand the concepts or to solve the problem? What are the learning issues?

After answering the above questions for this part of the case, go to Part Five.

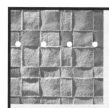 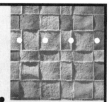

Case Study 8A • Part Five

Janice Bryan Moves to the Mountains

Conclusion

Three months later, on one of her regular visits to the Arnett family, Janice was pleased to learn that Mrs. Arnett was continuing to take her medication as prescribed.

Dave, Mrs. Arnett's son, told Janice that he had been watching some of the television programs about TB that the health department had sponsored.

"You know, it might not be a bad idea for us to get those skin tests you told us about," he said. "We would also like to know more about the shots you said the baby needed."

Thoughts & Notes

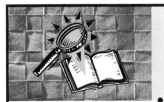 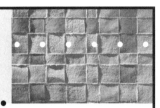

Case Analysis
Janice Bryan Moves to the Mountains

1. What are the concepts covered in the case?

2. What do you know about the case? What actual information do you have?

3. What are your provisional hypotheses?

4. What do you need to know to better understand the concepts or to solve the problem? What are the learning issues?

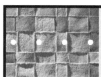 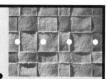

Case Study 8B • Part One
Rural Home Health Care

Case Material

Connie Posney, RN, BSN, is a home health nurse working in a rural county. The nearest city is about 115 miles to the north.

Connie received a referral to visit George Barnett, an 85-year-old patient in the end stages of Alzheimer's disease. When she called to arrange the visit, Connie learned that Mr. Barnett's daughter, 57-year-old Louise, is the primary caregiver. Other family members are Louise's husband, Al; and their son, Michael. All of the other family members have moved out of the region.

The family physician, Dr. Boggs, recently put Mr. Barnett on a new and complicated medication regimen. Connie learned that Medicare would allow three reimbursed visits to this family. As she prepared for the first visit, Connie wondered how best to teach the family in this short time.

The next day was her first visit. Connie introduced herself and asked Louise how she and Mr. Barnett were doing.

"I don't know if I can hang on much longer," Louise said, becoming tearful. "He needs so much care! I have to bathe him, feed him, dress him, and he doesn't even know who I am! A lot of times he tries to hit me.

"Now, Dr. Boggs has put him on all of these new medicines that I don't know what to do with. And anyway, Dad doesn't like to take pills and fights me when I try to get him to swallow them. I'm just at my wit's end, and there's no one to help me. The sitter refused to come back after the first week. I haven't been to church in 6 months, and I'm about to lose my job. I feel like I'm going crazy."

Connie calmed Louise and said, "I know you are feeling helpless and overwhelmed. Let's sit down and see if we can come up with some ideas to help you."

Thoughts & Notes

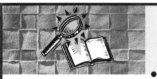 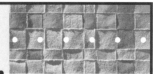

Case Analysis
Rural Home Health Care

1. What are the concepts covered in the case?

2. What do you know about the case? What actual information do you have?

3. What are your provisional hypotheses?

4. What do you need to know to better understand the concepts or to solve the problem? What are the learning issues?

After answering the above questions for this part of the case, go to Part Two.

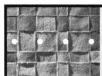

Case Study 8B • Part Two
Rural Home Health Care

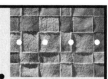

Case Material

Back at the office, Connie approached her supervisor, Todd Durham. "I need to talk with you about the visit I just made to the Barnett family," she said.

"Louise, the caregiver for Mr. Barnett, is feeling overwhelmed with the care of her father and all of her other responsibilities. Right now she is only able to process small amounts of information. The medication regimen alone would take more than three visits for her to understand. What is the possibility of doing three extra visits at no charge? We have done it in the past."

Todd paused for a moment and then said, "Connie, we have such a high caseload that we can't do any no-charge visits right now. And since our Medicare reimbursement rate is lower here than in urban areas, we're having a difficult time meeting our budget. Let's think about other ways to meet the needs of this family."

Thoughts & Notes

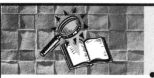
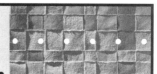

Case Analysis

Rural Home Health Care

1. What are the concepts covered in the case?

2. What do you know about the case? What actual information do you have?

3. What are your provisional hypotheses?

4. What do you need to know to better understand the concepts or to solve the problem? What are the learning issues?

After answering the above questions for this part of the case, go to Part Three.

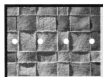 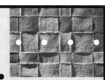

Case Study 8B • Part Three
Rural Home Health Care

Case Material

Todd went to Barb Johnson, the agency coordinator. "Barb, a situation has arisen involving George Barnett, which I believe should be addressed by the management staff. Do you think it would be possible to do this?"

"Tell me more," Barb said. "What particular issues of the case do you think need to be addressed by the team?"

"Mr. Barnett has extensive teaching needs, but is only allowed three reimbursed visits," Todd responded. "Do you think we could look into the Medicare Waiver Program? I'm also concerned about patient's rights issues and the possibility of abandonment. We need to look at our internal policy revisions that address reimbursement issues.

"I'm also concerned about the primary caregiver, Louise, who seems to be on the verge of a breakdown. We need to find assistance for her from the community. Sue Williams, our case manager, should be able to help us with this."

Barb suggested they hold a team meeting to discuss these problems.

Thoughts & Notes

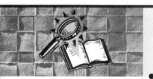 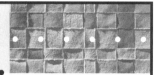

Case Analysis

Rural Home Health Care

1. What are the concepts covered in the case?

2. What do you know about the case? What actual information do you have?

3. What are your provisional hypotheses?

4. What do you need to know to better understand the concepts or to solve the problem? What are the learning issues?

After answering the above questions for this part of the case, go to Part Four.

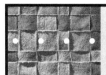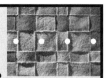

Case Study 8B • Part Four
Rural Home Health Care

Conclusion

After the team meeting to discuss the Barnetts' situation, Connie was able to contact the HMO case manager. He agreed to an additional four home visits.

Mr. Barnett was referred to the home- and community-based waiver program for elder care and respite services. Louise was referred to an Alzheimer's support group, which she attends twice a week. At her latest home visit, Louise told Connie things were getting better.

"I can handle the medicines," Louise said. "And now that Dad goes to the day-care center, I can go to work and don't have to worry about losing my job. Living with Dad's disease is still hard, but I'm learning that there are people out there who will give me help when I need it."

· · · · · Thoughts & Notes · · · · ·

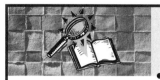
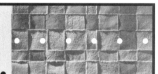

Case Analysis
Rural Home Health Care

1. What are the concepts covered in the case?

2. What do you know about the case? What actual information do you have?

3. What are your provisional hypotheses?

4. What do you need to know to better understand the concepts or to solve the problem? What are the learning issues?

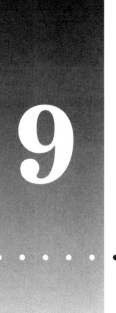

9 Nursing Case Management and Program Management

Juliann G. Sebastian

The cases in this chapter examine professional and advanced practice nursing roles in case management as part of community health nursing practice and program planning and management. The four case studies will stimulate continued learning about the major health problems in a given state or province and how they relate to national health goals. Whether a nurse lives in the United States or Canada, it is important to identify the major sources of information about the epidemiology of local health problems and how they compare with regional and national trends. Professional nurses need this type of data to develop health programs in partnership with community members.

The chapter also explores strategies for working with the community. Health professionals know that it is imperative to work in partnership with community members to identify health problems of greatest concern; identify community strengths, resources, and assets; and work collaboratively in designing health programs best-suited to local circumstances.

The cases also deal with fiscal issues and nursing informatics, areas essential to creating and supporting the context within which community health nursing occurs. Case Study 9A, Nursing Care Management at Monolith, and Case Study 9B, Cost of Nursing, emphasize the economic context within which community health nursing is practiced.

Case Study 9C, Dierdre Hopkins, and Case Study 9D, Trish Samuels and the Community Nursing Center, examine the role of public health within a managed care environment. The changing nature of this role means that nurses should be involved in policy debates about the optimal strategies for promoting and maintaining the health of the public. The student should read broadly and look closely for any learning issues in these cases to examine how wider sociopolitical issues influence direct provision of care.

Resources

Electronic Resources:

1. Search the Internet for sites related to nursing case management and managed care. Critique the information you find on these sites for its applicability to these cases. Do the sites include references to credible research to support the data or recommendations?
2. Identify Internet databases that describe the incidence and prevalence of the major chronic diseases in your state. Check the home pages for Medicare and Medicaid (http://www.fedstats.gov/index20.html) to determine the average cost of caring for people with these chronic health problems. How would you estimate the personal cost to people with chronic illnesses in terms of diminished quality of life and lost productivity?
3. Web sites

Healthy Cities USA	http://www.who.dk/tech/hcp/index.htm
World Health Organization	http://www.who.ch/
Joint Commission on Accreditation of Healthcare Organizations (JCAHO)	http://www.jcaho.org
Links to JCAHO health organizations	http://www.jcaho.org/link_frm.htm
American Heart Association	http://www.amhrt.org
American Cancer Association	http://www.cancer.org
National Institutes of Health (NIH)	http://www.nih.gov
Agency for Health Care Policy and Research	http://www.ahcpr.gov
Health Services Technology Assessment Text (an NIH service)	http://text.nlm.nih.gov/

People Resources:

1. Interview nurses in your community who work in case management roles to find out what models of nursing case management they use.
2. Interview administrators in managed care organizations to learn their perspectives on the major issues in providing a seamless continuum of care for populations with chronic illness.
3. Interview community leaders to determine what they believe are the major health needs and assets in your community.
4. Interview nurse leaders from the local health department and from a local primary care clinic.
5. Contact either a local business leader or the school of business at a nearby university to discuss the impact of the increasingly diverse workforce on organizational culture. Interview a faculty member in the school of business on what is meant by organizational development.

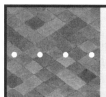 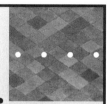

Case Study 9A • Part One
Nursing Care Management at Monolith

Case Material

Carolyn Smeltzer, MSN, RN, is developing a nursing care management program for a major managed care network in a midwestern state. The company for which she works, Monolith, has traditionally employed clerical staff to do a utilization review type of case management. Recently, the chief executive officer (CEO) has begun to think that it is important to add a clinician to do case management.

In thinking about the new program she is developing, Carolyn realizes that she needs to identify the scope of the responsibilities inherent in such a role. She decides to interview some key people in order to better understand it.

Carolyn wishes to contrast the role in the community with that of an institutionally based care manager. She is particularly interested in focusing on key target populations within the state. Recognizing that this care management program needs to work with the most common chronic diseases in the population, she chooses an epidemiological approach to collect and analyze data.

Thoughts & Notes

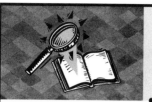
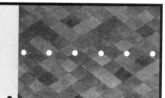

Case Analysis
Nursing Care Management at Monolith

1. What are the concepts covered in the case?

2. What do you know about the case? What actual information do you have?

3. What are your provisional hypotheses?

4. What do you need to know to better understand the concepts or to solve the problem? What are the learning issues?

After answering the above questions for this part of the case, go to Part Two.

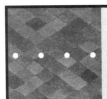 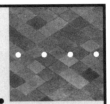

Case Study 9A • Part Two
Nursing Care Management at Monolith

Case Material

Carolyn knows that some of the Monolith client groups participate in managed care plans, whereas others are still members of indemnity plans. However, she is not familiar with the reasons why one would choose between indemnity and managed care plans. Like everyone else at Monolith, she is acutely aware that Medicaid is shifting all of its enrollees to managed care plans and that Medicare is likely to follow in the future.

Other changes are likely to occur within the state as well that have everyone in Monolith management concerned. A group of legislators has proposed that health insurance plans be required to adopt a community rating system and drop their prior illness exclusions. Steve Cohen, Monolith CEO, commented on his worry that the company might be experiencing some adverse selection in its managed care plan. Given the demographic make-up and risk profile of the population, he wished the company could add questions to its screening criteria for enrollees.

"Why is he acting as if this is more important for a managed care plan?" Carolyn wonders.

She is also puzzled by Steve's remark about needing to move to a community rating system. He had shared with her his worry that they would not be able to keep costs low enough to compete for contracts with some of the larger employers in the area, particularly those that were self-insured. ACME Manufacturing, one of the largest employers in the state, was already trying to negotiate sharply discounted rates.

Thoughts & Notes

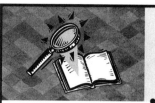

Case Analysis
Nursing Care Management at Monolith

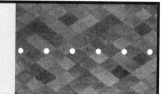

1. What are the concepts covered in the case?

2. What do you know about the case? What actual information do you have?

3. What are your provisional hypotheses?

4. What do you need to know to better understand the concepts or to solve the problem? What are the learning issues?

After answering the above questions for this part of the case, go to Part Three.

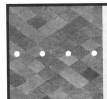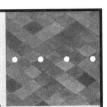

Case Study 9A • Part Three
Nursing Care Management at Monolith

Case Material

Several weeks after Carolyn began working on developing her care management program, she called her colleague, John Williams. John works as a nurse care manager in an integrated service network in Minnesota.

"John, I need to talk with you about your program and how you are organized within your system," Carolyn began.

"The vice president for clinical services told me to be sure to design my program so it accounts for the fact that we are vertically integrated. She also said I need to take into account the alliances we are developing with other systems. She said something about the impact that the differences between vertical and horizontal integration might have on the way I design this program.

"I am very confused about this and would appreciate your advice. To tell you the truth, this seems to be a bit out of my realm as a care manager. I think the vice president should probably be discussing these things with someone in management, instead of with me."

"I will be glad to discuss this with you," John said. "First, tell me what you have done so far in terms of developing your program."

"I am starting with a program focused on people who experience back injuries," Carolyn said. "The state is going to contract with us to begin doing some Workers' Compensation case management, so I have to develop a plan for that group. After I get an idea as to how well that is working, I am probably going to move to one of the top diagnosis-related group (DRG) categories."

Thoughts & Notes

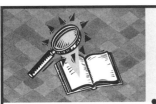

Case Analysis
Nursing Care Management at Monolith

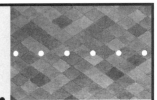

1. What are the concepts covered in the case?

2. What do you know about the case? What actual information do you have?

3. What are your provisional hypotheses?

4. What do you need to know to better understand the concepts or to solve the problem? What are the learning issues?

After answering the above questions for this part of the case, go to Part Four.

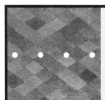
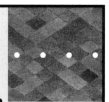

Case Study 9A • Part Four
Nursing Care Management at Monolith

Case Material

Carolyn's Workers' Compensation case management program had been in effect for 6 months. She was pleased with the relationships she had developed with the people at the state level and felt that her clients were satisfied with the help she was providing in coordinating the services they needed. However, there were frustrations, too.

She was having difficulty finding the right people with whom to work in the various health care agencies she had contacted, and there was a lack of communication across agencies. She had spoken with some wonderful clinicians, but overall she was running into numerous barriers in obtaining information, getting through to people who could make clinical decisions, and collaborating with clinicians. Carolyn was quite concerned about developing strong collaborative relationships with people in other agencies—not only clinicians, but also receptionists, administrators, financial staff, and others.

She was also having problems with the clinical pathways. Few clients could be managed effectively with the pathways, in large part because of coordination difficulties across agencies.

She called her friend John again. He suggested that she organize an advisory council for her program. "Where should I begin?" Carolyn wondered.

Thoughts & Notes

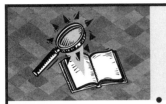

Case Analysis
Nursing Care Management
at Monolith

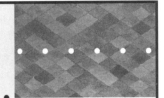

1. What are the concepts covered in the case?

2. What do you know about the case? What actual information do you have?

3. What are your provisional hypotheses?

4. What do you need to know to better understand the concepts or to solve the problem? What are the learning issues?

After answering the above questions for this part of the case, go to Part Five.

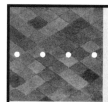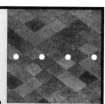

Case Study 9A • Part Five

Nursing Care Management at Monolith

Conclusion

"Did you ever think this program would develop like it has?" Yolanda Garcia smiled as she and Carolyn discussed the new program over a cup of coffee.

"No," Carolyn admitted. "I am delighted that it has taken on these new dimensions, but I certainly never would have predicted it."

What had begun as a nursing care management program for people who had filed Workers' Compensation claims for back injuries had become the "Healthy Workers" program. Based on feedback from the new Community Advisory Council, the program was expanded from its focus on tertiary prevention with people who had already suffered injuries to include primary and secondary preventive services as well. Monolith no longer contracted solely with the Workers' Compensation program, but now held contracts with numerous businesses.

As managed care saturation had increased in the community, health care organizations had begun taking a more proactive approach to improving community health. They were now partnering with the local health department and community members to determine the roles that Monolith could play in furthering community health.

"I don't know where we will go from here," mused Carolyn, "but I am excited about our current direction."

Thoughts & Notes

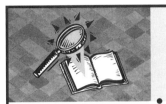

Case Analysis
Nursing Care Management at Monolith

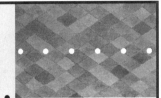

1. What are the concepts covered in the case?

2. What do you know about the case? What actual information do you have?

3. What are your provisional hypotheses?

4. What do you need to know to better understand the concepts or to solve the problem? What are the learning issues?

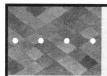 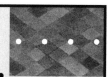

Case Study 9B • Part One
Cost of Nursing

Case Material

"How can I be asked to reduce the cost of providing care for our congestive heart failure (CHF) clients when I don't even know what it costs to provide their care?"

Betty Sowell, BSN, is one of the case managers at Good Samaritan Health System (GSHS). Good Samaritan is a large, vertically integrated system that includes two primary care clinics, a 300-bed hospital, a home health agency, and a total of 100 long-term care beds located in two nursing homes.

Good Samaritan had put a case management program in place earlier in the year to begin following high-risk, high-volume target populations through the system. The program was supposed to focus on health promotion and illness prevention within the target populations. Approximately 20% of the insured population in Good Samaritan's market is covered by managed care plans, but that percentage is beginning to rise rapidly.

Betty and the three other nurse case managers refining the program have been concerned about tracking costs since the beginning. Betty works primarily with the Cardiovascular Services Product Line. She has just received a memo from Donna Javitt, MSN, director of the Cardiovascular Services Product Line, asking her to devise a strategy for reducing the costs of the CHF diagnosis-related group (DRG). She wants Betty to present her plan at the Product Line team meeting scheduled later in the month.

Betty looked at her colleagues. "How do you think I should go about responding to Donna's request?" she asked.

• • • • • • *Thoughts & Notes* • • • • • •

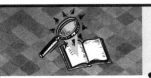

Case Analysis
Cost of Nursing

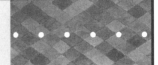

1. What are the concepts covered in this case?

2. What do you know about the case? What actual information do you have?

3. What are your provisional hypotheses?

4. What do you need to know to better understand the concepts or to solve the problem? What are the learning issues?

After answering the above questions for this part of the case, go to Part Two.

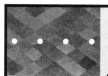 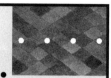

Case Study 9B • Part Two
Cost of Nursing

Case Material

The nurse case managers met to discuss Betty's dilemma. "This sounds like it could be a pretty big project," said Jerry Hamilton, MSN, RN. Jerry specializes in trauma and catastrophic injury cases. "Why don't you break this down into more manageable pieces?

"For example, you could start by trying to find out how much it costs, on average, to provide care for a CHF patient in the hospital. Then you could talk with one of the primary care clinics about their usual cost of caring for these patients. Finally, you could call Gina Hartley over at home health and find out what their costs are for these patients."

"Well, that is a good idea, Jerry, but I am not quite sure where I will find that information," Betty said doubtfully. "I think I could call the chief financial officer and get the standard charges from each of those areas. But when it comes to the actual costs, it seems like such a complicated issue.

"Let's talk about your suggestion some more," she said. "I could really use some ideas."

Thoughts & Notes

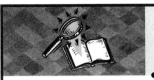 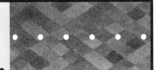

Case Analysis
Cost of Nursing

1. What are the concepts covered in this case?

2. What do you know about the case? What actual information do you have?

3. What are your provisional hypotheses?

4. What do you need to know to better understand the concepts or to solve the problem? What are the learning issues?

After answering the above questions for this part of the case, go to Part Three.

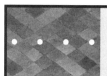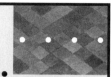

Case Study 9B • Part Three
Cost of Nursing

Case Material

"Could you check with the nursing department of the GSHS hospital to find out how much nursing care these patients require, using the Patient Classification System?" Jerry suggested. "That way, you could calculate the total costs of nursing care based on the Relative Value Units required by CHF patients."

Betty thought for a few moments. That could be a really good strategy, she decided. Even though that would not tell her the total costs of caring for this population of patients, it would give her a measure of costs based on the amount of nursing resources they required. This would give her a severity-adjusted way of analyzing that DRG.

"You know, this whole project might be very helpful for us," Jerry went on. "It will give us a chance to think about how we would price nursing care management services for CHF patients for any number of managed care contracts."

Thoughts & Notes

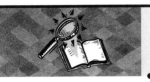

Case Analysis
Cost of Nursing

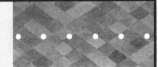

1. What are the concepts covered in this case?

2. What do you know about the case? What actual information do you have?

3. What are your provisional hypotheses?

4. What do you need to know to better understand the concepts or to solve the problem? What are the learning issues?

After answering the above questions for this part of the case, go to Part Four.

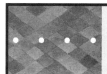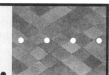

Case Study 9B • Part Four
Cost of Nursing

Case Material

As Betty investigated the Patient Classification System in use at the GSHS hospital, she realized that it did not provide a very clear picture of clients' nursing resource needs. It did not do a very good job of predicting nursing needs during an individual's hospitalization, nor did it help in any way to predict clients' nursing resource needs in the clinic setting or in home health.

What was more, Betty learned, the system did not provide any information about the kinds of health promotion and illness prevention services nurse care managers could offer, since it was geared only toward clients' illness experience.

"How would I go about determining the full extent of nursing resources these clients require?" she wondered.

Thoughts & Notes

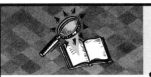 **Case Analysis**
Cost of Nursing

1. What are the concepts covered in this case?

2. What do you know about the case? What actual information do you have?

3. What are your provisional hypotheses?

4. What do you need to know to better understand the concepts or to solve the problem? What are the learning issues?

After answering the above questions for this part of the case, go to Part Five.

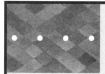 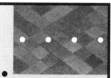

Case Study 9B • Part Five
Cost of Nursing

Conclusion

Betty brought the matter up with Donna Javitt later that week.

"I think you have raised a good issue," Donna said. "Why don't we think about limiting your plan to those clients who have recently been discharged from the hospital?

"We could focus on preventing readmissions and on enhancing their quality of life. That way, you could limit your analysis and planning to the period following discharge from the hospital and focus on the problems, interventions, and outcomes that are appropriate for that point. I think we have probably reduced the costs associated with length of stay about as much as we can. This is the point in the service continuum that we really need to concentrate on, anyway."

"Good idea," said Betty. "I have been doing some reading about linking nursing problems with ICD-9 (International Classification of Diseases-ninth revision) codes and linking nursing interventions with CPT (Current Procedural Terminology) codes. Perhaps I could develop a data base that would link these elements of clients' nursing resource utilization and track costs that way. Then I could work with the clinics and the home health agency to plan programming that would really help these folks with CHF stay healthier."

"Sounds like a great place to begin," Donna said.

Thoughts & Notes

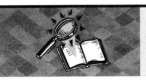

1. What are the concepts covered in this case?

2. What do you know about the case? What actual information do you have?

3. What are your provisional hypotheses?

4. What do you need to know to better understand the concepts or to solve the problem? What are the learning issues?

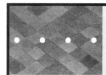 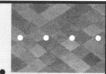

Case Study 9C • Part One
Dierdre Hopkins

Case Material

Dierdre looked out at the mountains past the city. She had just completed a very full day at a conference on primary health care and was excited about having many ideas for a community health center.

She had heard speakers from around the country describe community health centers that really operationalized the idea of primary health care and were truly responsive to the local cultures in their communities. She had also heard one speaker talk about the Healthy Cities movement, and was mulling over the whole idea of a Healthy City.

"I wonder how much of this we can put in place in Clover City?" she thought. "I know we certainly have plenty of people at the health department that would be interested in these ideas. But the key is to involve other people as well."

LaToya Trimble came over and sat down, and Dierdre began sharing some of her thoughts.

"What I am excited about are the ideas about PATCH (Planned Approach to Community Health) and APEXPH (Assessment Protocol for Excellence in Public Health) that one of the speakers described," LaToya said. "However, none of the people at our place are familiar with those ideas. It would take some education to get everyone on board."

Thoughts & Notes

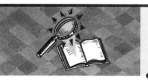

Case Analysis
Dierdre Hopkins

1. What are the concepts covered in this case?

2. What do you know about the case? What actual information do you have?

3. What are your provisional hypotheses?

4. What do you need to know to better understand the concepts or to solve the problem? What are the learning issues?

After answering the above questions for this part of the case, go to Part Two.

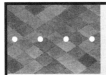
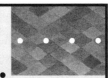

Case Study 9C • Part Two
Dierdre Hopkins

Case Material

After Dierdre returned home, she contacted her colleague, Joe Ross. Joe is the director of Alpha Health Center, a Section 330 community health clinic in another state. She wanted to talk with him about the kinds of services his clinic provides and the volume and mix of patients they serve.

Dierdre had spoken with LaToya at some length during the conference, and came away more convinced than ever that she needed to work with the Clover City Health Department staff to plan a community health clinic. She was not sure if it would be a good idea to try to get Section 330 funding, but did think she wanted to involve the community in planning the clinic.

Dierdre knows that Joe has been with Alpha since its beginning, 15 years ago. "Joe, what did you find to be the most important step in planning your clinic?" she asked.

"I think one critical step is to figure out what types of needs the community has, and then determine what services you can provide to meet those needs." he said.

"We have found that we are seeing more and more patients with hypertension and diabetes. If you want, I can send you a printout of our last 5 years of service data to show you how many visits have been coded with these two diagnoses. That may give you some ideas."

"Thanks so much, Joe." Dierdre said.

· · · · · · Thoughts & Notes · · · · · ·

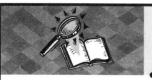

Case Analysis
Dierdre Hopkins

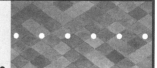

1. What are the concepts covered in this case?

2. What do you know about the case? What actual information do you have?

3. What are your provisional hypotheses?

4. What do you need to know to better understand the concepts or to solve the problem? What are the learning issues?

After answering the above questions for this part of the case, go to Part Three.

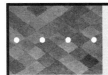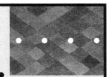

Case Study 9C • Part Three
Dierdre Hopkins

Case Material

As Dierdre thought through the possibilities for planning a community health clinic, she became convinced that such a clinic needed to include services related to the preconditions for health.

She contacted Saundra Talcott, MSW, the County Commissioner for Social Services. Saundra was very interested, but worried about the potential for conflicting organizational cultures if social work and primary care clinic staffs were mixed.

"The social workers in my department are not medical social workers," Saundra said. "They are more accustomed to handling food stamps and welfare applications than working with health-related issues. I think we may have to do some organizational development to help both groups work as a team."

"That's a great idea," agreed Dierdre. "If we go that route, I think we should add some diversity training. As long as we are starting something from the ground up, we should really focus on creating a warm and welcoming environment. We have such a large Asian population here in Clover City that we should make sure that everything we do is culturally competent."

Thoughts & Notes

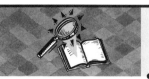

Case Analysis
Dierdre Hopkins

1. What are the concepts covered in this case?

2. What do you know about the case? What actual information do you have?

3. What are your provisional hypotheses?

4. What do you need to know to better understand the concepts or to solve the problem? What are the learning issues?

After answering the above questions for this part of the case, go to Part Four.

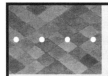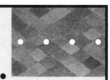

Case Study 9C • Part Four
Dierdre Hopkins

Conclusion

Dierdre and Saundra worked together for a year on planning the new clinic. They established a clinic task force that fully participated in the needs assessment and planning stages. The task force included members from the health department and the social service department staffs, as well as leaders from the local Asian community.

The task force ran into some difficulties in planning ways to evaluate the effectiveness of the clinic, however. Their initial plan was to distribute patient satisfaction surveys to every tenth patient served throughout Year One, then randomly select patients on a quarterly basis.

Several members of the task force raised questions about the usefulness of this approach. They questioned whether the data would really help them evaluate important questions about the clinic's effectiveness. Further, they were concerned about the patients' comfort with written surveys, and the logistics of getting the surveys back.

"You know, I think we should really spend our time investigating ways to develop computerized patient records and link those records with the overall health department clinical information system," Wan Lu said. Ms. Lu was one of the key Asian leaders participating on the task force. "Isn't it most important that we show that we have helped people improve their health?"

Wan's challenging questions led the task force to revise their evaluation plan to include measurement of selected clinical outcomes, and begin working with the health department to investigate the feasibility of computerized patient records.

Dierdre was pleased that a comprehensive community health clinic was scheduled to open later in the year in an area of the city with a large Asian population.

Thoughts & Notes

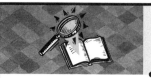

Case Analysis
Dierdre Hopkins

1. What are the concepts covered in this case?

2. What do you know about the case? What actual information do you have?

3. What are your provisional hypotheses?

4. What do you need to know to better understand the concepts or to solve the problem? What are the learning issues?

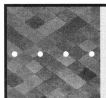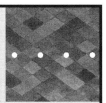

Case Study 9D • Part One
Trish Samuels and the Community Nursing Center

Case Material

Trish Samuels closed the cover of the proposal and wondered how she would develop the marketing plan that Angela had requested.

The Henderson Community Nursing Center, where Trish was employed, had submitted a proposal to the state to fund a comprehensive human immunodeficiency virus (HIV) prevention, treatment, and care management (PTCM) program. The goals of the PTCM program were broad. Trish was concerned about the best way to develop the marketing plan, given the overall scope of the program.

The objectives were to:

1. Reduce the incidence of HIV infection in the area served by the Henderson Community Nursing Center by 10% in 3 years by providing preventive education to the community.
2. Help HIV-positive individuals obtain the necessary treatment to delay the onset of symptoms.
3. Assist people with acquired immunodeficiency syndrome (AIDS) in the management of symptoms.
4. Link people with AIDS to the necessary services through a care management program.

Angela Murray, RN, MSN, was the director of the Nursing Center. She believed strongly in illness prevention and generally favored comprehensive programs. However, Trish thought that marketing such a program might be tricky.

• • • • • Thoughts & Notes • • • • •

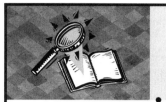 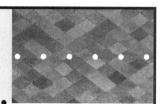

Case Analysis
Trish Samuels and the Community Nursing Center

1. What are the concepts covered in this case?

2. What do you know about the case? What actual information do you have?

3. What are your provisional hypotheses?

4. What do you need to know to better understand the concepts or to solve the problem? What are the learning issues?

After answering the above questions for this part of the case, go to Part Two.

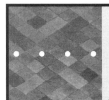 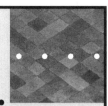

Case Study 9D • Part Two

Trish Samuels and the Community Nursing Center

Case Material

The proposal for the HIV PTCM program was rejected, primarily because the reviewers thought that the program evaluation had not been sufficiently well planned. In fact, little was in the proposal about evaluation, except one paragraph. The next proposal submission date was 2 months away, so Angela wanted to resubmit the proposal after strengthening the evaluation portion.

Trish had done a good job designing a plan to market the program to the community, and Angela thought she would be the ideal person to coordinate the development of an evaluation plan. She called Trish into her office one afternoon to discuss it.

"Trish, I know you are as disappointed as I am about this proposal," Angela said. "However, the reviewers were right on target. Our evaluation plan was inadequate. I really want to resubmit the proposal, though. We need this program in our community, and we just can't let one setback stop us. Would you take on the task of developing the evaluation plan?

"I could ask Joe and Marilyn to help you, and give you some time away from your usual responsibilities to work on this. If you are willing, I would like to see some initial ideas in a week, and then we should look at a complete draft 3 weeks from now. The final plan won't need to be approved until 6 weeks from today."

"Yes, I think we have to move ahead," Trish agreed. "I have a number of things I am working on right now, but I do appreciate your offer of help and would be happy to spearhead the development of the evaluation plan."

"Good," said Angela. "The first thing I think you should determine are the major questions the evaluation should focus on. Then I suggest that you develop drafts of one or two data collection instruments to help us get a feel for the kind of data we will need and the problems we might run into in getting that data. Don't spend too long on these instruments, though, because we will need to spend a lot more time figuring out exactly what data to collect to answer the evaluation questions. Could you get back to me with these things next Monday?"

"Yes, I can do that," Trish said.

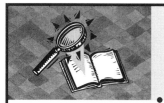

Case Analysis
Trish Samuels and the Community Nursing Center

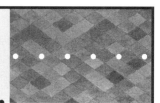

1. What are the concepts covered in this case?

2. What do you know about the case? What actual information do you have?

3. What are your provisional hypotheses?

4. What do you need to know to better understand the concepts or to solve the problem? What are the learning issues?

After answering the above questions for this part of the case, go to Part Three.

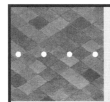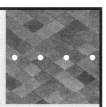

Case Study 9D • Part Three
Trish Samuels and the Community Nursing Center

Case Material

Trish decided to begin her evaluation plan by focusing on the third program goal: to assist people with AIDS in the management of symptoms.

She began by asking the following question: "Did people with AIDS who participated in the program experience fewer problems with symptomatology than people who did not participate in the program?"

As Trish began considering the issues she would have to deal with in the evaluation, she wondered what standards would be appropriate to use in answering this question. Further, as she reflected on the question, she began to think that it would be very difficult to get data on people with AIDS who were not in the program.

"How can we demonstrate whether the program achieves this goal or not?" Trish wondered.

Thoughts & Notes

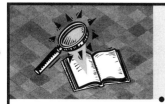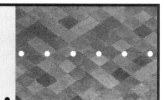

Case Analysis
Trish Samuels and the Community Nursing Center

1. What are the concepts covered in this case?

2. What do you know about the case? What actual information do you have?

3. What are your provisional hypotheses?

4. What do you need to know to better understand the concepts or to solve the problem? What are the learning issues?

After answering the above questions for this part of the case, go to Part Four.

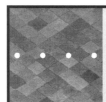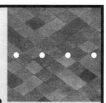

Case Study 9D • Part Four
Trish Samuels and the Community Nursing Center

Case Material

Trish conducted a literature review to determine what experiences other programs had been having in helping people with AIDS manage their symptoms.

"Look at this," she told Angela. "There is a program in California that demonstrated a 10% improvement in pain management after a 5-week pain management program, and the findings were statistically significant. They only had 30 patients in the program. But still, that is a really remarkable result. Maybe we should adopt their program."

"Maybe so," Angela said, "but a 10% improvement doesn't seem like much. How much did their program cost? Does the report say anything about how the participants felt about it?"

• • • • • Thoughts & Notes • • • • •

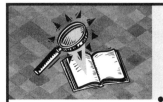
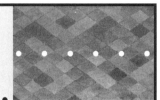

Case Analysis
Trish Samuels and the Community Nursing Center

1. What are the concepts covered in this case?

2. What do you know about the case? What actual information do you have?

3. What are your provisional hypotheses?

4. What do you need to know to better understand the concepts or to solve the problem? What are the learning issues?

After answering the above questions for this part of the case, go to Part Five.

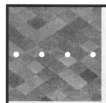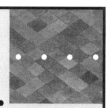

Case Study 9D • Part Five
Trish Samuels and the Community Nursing Center

Conclusion

Trish presented her draft evaluation plan for the HIV PCTM program to Angela.

"Wonderful!," Angela said. "Tell me, what are the highlights of this plan?"

"Well, I have broken the plan down into four major sections to correspond to the four overall program goals," Trish said. "We have baseline data on the incidence of HIV infection from our needs assessment, so the first goal is to keep track of that data so we can identify trends and compare the incidence rate with baseline at the end of 3 years.

"For the second goal, I have developed a questionnaire to ask our HIV-positive clients which of the major symptoms they are experiencing upon admission to the program. I have also included a checklist for case managers to use to indicate which referrals they make for their clients, what the outcomes of follow-up are, and when symptoms appear. We can compare the timing of the onset of symptoms with the data being reported in the literature to get an idea of the effectiveness of our referrals."

Angela looked impressed. Trish went on. "We will need to develop symptom management protocols with the case managers. We also need to go ahead and get the physicians involved in the process.

"In addition to the medically oriented protocols, I think we should use the Nursing Interventions Classification to help us track the interventions we use. I have developed a template of a checklist that we might use to do the tracking on client symptoms using the Nursing Minimum Data Set and the North American Nursing Diagnoses. You will find a second template for use in tracking the therapeutic nursing interventions. Of course, the actual protocols will determine the final format of these data collection tools. We should pilot these to make sure they are valid and reliable.

"Finally, I recommend similar evaluation procedures for the fourth goal. I want to ask your opinion about whether to analyze some of this data midway through the 3-year project. I think this would be helpful because we could go ahead and revise anything that doesn't seem to be working. Also, I would like to discuss the possibility of organizing meetings once a year between the case managers and providers out in the community to evaluate how the referral linkages are working."

"Well," said Angela, "you have clearly done a lot of work. I will read your plan and get back to you. Thank you for such great work."

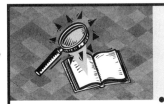 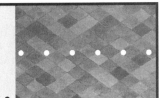

Case Analysis
Trish Samuels and the Community Nursing Center

1. What are the concepts covered in this case?

2. What do you know about the case? What actual information do you have?

3. What are your provisional hypotheses?

4. What do you need to know to better understand the concepts or to solve the problem? What are the learning issues?

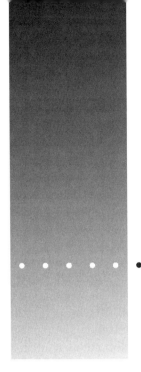

References
and Resources

The citations for Chapters 1-3 are referred to in the text for those chapters. Materials listed for Chapters 4-9 are suggested resources for students wishing to learn more about issues raised in the case studies.

Chapters 1-3

Barrows, H.S. (1988). *The tutorial process*. Springfield, IL: Southern Illinois University School of Medicine.

Barrows, H., & Feltovich, P.J. (1987). The clinical reasoning process. *Medical Education, 21*(2), 86-91.

Brookfield, S.D. (1995). *Becoming a critically reflective teacher*. San Francisco: Jossey-Bass.

Driscoll, J. (1994). Reflective practice for practise. *Senior Nurse, 14*(1), 47-50.

Joyce, L., & Weil, M. (1986). *Models of teaching*. New Jersey: Prentice-Hall.

King, M.G., Sebastian, J.G., Stanhope, M.K., & Hickman, J.J. (1997). Using problem-based learning to prepare advanced practice community health nurses for the 21st Century. *Family and Community Health, 20*(1), 29-39.

Nash, P. (1994). Problem-based learning. Presented January 10, 1994, at the Faculty Development Workshop, University of Kentucky College of Nursing, Lexington, Kentucky.

Schon, D. (1983). *The reflective practitioner*. New York: Basic Books.

Townsend, J. (1990). Curriculum design. *Nursing Times, 86*(18), 60-62.

Waterman, R., & Butler, C. (1985). Curriculum: Problems to stimulate learning. In A. Kaufman (Ed.), *Implementing problem-based medical education*. New York: Springer.

Chapter 4

Aiken, L.H., & Salmon, M.E. (1994). Health care workforce priorities: What nursing should do now. *Inquiry, 31*(3), 318-329.

American Nurses Association. (1985). *Standards of community health nursing practice.* Kansas City, MO: ANA.

American Public Health Association. (1997). *The definition and role of public health nursing in the delivery of health care.* Washington, DC: APHA.

American Public Health Association & National Association of County Health Officials. (1991). *APEXPH: Assessment protocol for excellence in public health.* Washington, DC: NACHO.

Aroskar, M.A. (1989). Community health nurses: Their most significant ethical decision-making problems. *Nursing Clinics of North America, 24*(4), 967-975.

Baldwin, J.H. (1995). Are we implementing community health promotion in nursing? *Public Health Nursing, 12*(3), 159-164.

Barger, S. (1991). The nursing center: A model for rural nursing practice. *Nursing and Health Care, 12*(6), 290-294.

Barger, S. (1991). Public health nursing partnership: Agencies and academe. *Nurse Educator, 16*(4), 16-8.

Dienemann, J. (1992). Designing a marketing plan that works. *Journal of Nursing Administration, 22*(1), 23-28.

Fenton, M.V., & Brykcznski, K.A. (1993). Qualitative distinctions and similarities in the practice of clinical nurse specialists and nurse practitioners. *Journal of Professional Nursing, 9*(6), 313-326.

Fenton, M.V., Rounds, L.R., & Anderson, E.T. (1991). Combining the role of the nurse practitioner and the community health nurse: An educational model for implementing community-based primary health care. *Journal of the American Academy of Nurse Practitioners, 3*(3), 99-105.

Griffith, H.M. (1993). Needed: A strong nursing position on preventive service. *Image, 25*(4), 272.

Hanric, A., Spross, J. & Hanson, C. (1996). *Advanced nursing practice: An integrated approach.* Philadelphia: Saunders.

Hanson, C. (1991). The 1990s and beyond: Determining the need for community health and primary care nurses for rural populations. *The Journal of Rural Health, 7*(1), 413-425.

Helvie, C.O. (1998). *Advanced nursing practice in the community.* Thousand Oaks, CA: Sage.

Institute of Medicine, Committee on the Future of Public Health. (1988). *The Future of Public Health.* Washington, DC: National Academy Press.

Jenkins, M. & Sullivan, M. (1994). Nurse practitioners and community health nurses: Clinical partnerships and future visions. *Nursing Clinics of North America, 29*(3), 459-470.

Josten, L., Clarke, P.N., Oswald, S., Stoskopf, C., & Shannon, M.D. (1995). Public health nursing education: Back to the future for public health sciences. *Family & Community Health, 18*(1), 36-48, 22.

Kelly, C., Cowell, J.M., & Stevens, R. (1997). Surveying public health nurses' continuing education needs: Collaboration of practice and academia, *Journal of Continuing Education in Nursing, 28*(3), 115-123.

King, P.M. (1994). Health promotion: The emerging frontier in nursing. *Journal of Advanced Practice Nursing, 29*(2), 209-218.

Lamb, G., Donaldson, N., & Kellogg, J. (1998). *Case management: A guide to strategic evaluation.* St. Louis: Mosby.

Lambert, V., & Lambert, C. (1996). Advanced practice nurses: Starting an independent practice. *Nursing Forum, 31*(1), 11-21.

Leigh, B. (1993). Case management in a health maintenance organization. *AAOHN Journal, 41*(4), 170-173.

Manion, J. (1991). Nurse entrepreneurs: The heroes of health care's future. *Nursing Outlook, 39*(1), 18-21.

Mason, D., Knight, K., Toughill, E., DeMaio, D., Beck, T., & Christopher, M.A. (1992). Promoting the community health clinical nurse specialist. *Clinical Nurse Specialist, 6*(1), 6-13.

May, K.M., Mendelson, C., & Ferketich, S. (1995). Community empowerment in rural health care. *Public Health Nursing, 12*(1), 25-30.

Micheels, T.A., Wheeler, L.M., & Hays, B.J. (1995). Linking quality and cost effectiveness: Case management by an advanced practice nurse. *Clinical Nurse Specialist, 9*(2), 107-111.

Monterio, L.A. (1985). Florence Nightingale on public health nursing. *American Journal of Public Health, 75*(2), 181-186.

Newman, M., Lamb, G.S., & Michaels, C. (1991). Nurse case management: The coming together of theory and practice. *Nursing and Health Care, 12*(8), 404-408.

Ponte, P.R., Higgins, J.M., James, J.R., Fay, M., & Madden, M.J. (1993). Development needs of advance practice nurses in a managed care environment. *Journal of Nursing Administration, 23*(11), 13-9.

Pearson, L. (1997). Annual update of how each state stands on legislative issues affecting advance nursing practice. *Journal of the American Academy of Nurse Practitioners, 21*(1), 10-70.

Rains, J.W., & Ray, D.W. (1995). Participatory action research for community health promotion. *Public Health Nursing, 12*(4), 256-261.

Rogers, M. (1991). Community-based nursing case management pays off. *Nursing Management, 22*(3), 31-34.

Selby, M., Riportella-Muller, R., Quade, D., Legault, C., & Salmon, M. (1990). Core curriculum for master's level community health nursing education: A comparison of the views of leaders in service and education. *Public Health Nursing, 7*(3), 150-160.

Stanhope, M., & Lancaster, J. (1996). *Community health nursing: Promoting the health of aggregates, families and individuals* (4th ed.). St. Louis: Mosby.

Turnock, B.J. (1997). *Public health: What it is and how it works.* Gaithersburg, MD: Aspen.

United States Department of Health & Human Services. (1991). *Healthy people 2000: national health promotion and disease prevention objectives.* (DHHS No. 91-50212). Washington, DC: U.S. Government Printing Office.

Williams, A. (1993). Steps to develop a working relationship: An evaluation of the community-based clinical nurse specialist. *Professional Nurse, 8*(12), 806, 808-10, 812.

Chapter 5

Benenson, A. (1995). *Control of communicable disease in man.* Washington, DC: American Public Health Association.

Brownson, R.C., Remington, P.L., & Davis, J.R. (Eds.). (1995). *Chronic disease epidemiology and control.* Washington, DC: American Public Health Association.

Centers for Disease Control. (1992). *Principles of epidemiology: Self-study course 3030G* (2nd ed.). Atlanta: CDC.

Stone, D.B., Armstrong, R.W., Macrina, D.M., & Pandau, J.W. (1996). *Introduction to epidemiology.* Madison, WI: Brown & Benchmark.

Timmreck, T.C. (1994). *Introduction to epidemiology.* Boston: Jones & Bartlett.

United States Department of Health & Human Services. (1991). *Healthy people 2000: National health promotion and disease prevention objectives.* (DHHS No. 91-50212). Washington, DC: U.S. Government Printing Office.

Valanis, B. (1992). *Epidemiology in nursing and health care.* Stamford, CT: Appleton & Lange.

Chapter 6

American Public Health Association & National Association of County Health officials. (1991). *APEXPH: Assessment protocol for excellence in public health.* Washington, DC: NACHO.

American Public Health Association. (1991). *Healthy communities 2000: Model standards* (3rd ed.). Washington, DC: U.S. Government Printing Office.

American Public Health Association & Centers for Disease Control and Prevention. (1993). *The guide to implementing model standards: Eleven steps toward a healthy community.* Washington, DC: APHA.

Anderson, E.T., & McFarlane, J.M. (1996). *Community as partner.* Philadelphia: Lippincott.

Bomar, P.J. (1989). *Nurses and family health promotion: Concepts, assessment, and interventions.* Philadelphia: W.B. Saunders.

Bracht, N. (1990). *Health promotion at the community level.* Thousand Oaks, CA: Sage.

Centers for Disease Control and Prevention. (1992) *PATCH: Planned approach to community health.* Atlanta: CDC.

Danielson, C.B., & Hamel-Bissell, B.P. (1993). *Families, health and illness.* St. Louis: Mosby.

Edelman, C.L., & Mandle, C.L. (1994). *Health promotion through the life span* (3rd ed.). St. Louis: Mosby.

Gilmore, G.D., & Campbell, M.D. (1996). *Needs assessment strategies for health education and health promotion* (2nd ed.). Madison, WI: Brown & Benchmark.

Green, L.W., & Kreuter, M.W. (1991). *Health promotion planning: An educational and environmental approach* (2nd ed.). Mountain View: Mayfield.

Miller, C.A., Moore, K.S., Richards, T.S., Monk, J.D. (1994) A proposed method for assessing the performance of local public health functions and practices. *American Journal of Public Health, 84*(11), 1743-1749.

Nasca, P.C. (1995) Public health assessment in the 1990s, (Editorial). *Journal of Public Health Management and Practice, 1*(2), vii-viii.

Pender, N.J. (1996). *Health promotion in nursing practice.* Stamford, CT: Appleton & Lange.

Richards, T.B., Rogers, J.J., Christenson, G.M., Miller, C.A., Gatewood, D.D., & Taylor, M.S. (1995). Assessing public health practice: Application of ten core function measures of community health in six states. *American Journal of Preventive Medicine, 11*(Suppl. 6): 36-40.

Rothman, J. (1987). Three models of community organization practice. In Cox, F. (Ed.), *Strategies of community organization* (pp. 3-26). Itasca, IL: Peacock.

United States Department of Health & Human Services. (1991). *Healthy people 2000: National health promotion and disease prevention objectives.* (DHHS No. 91-50212). Washington, DC: U.S. Government Printing Office.

United States Department of Health and Human Services. (1995). *Healthy people 2000: Midcourse review and 1995 revision.* Washington, DC: U.S. Government Printing Office.

Wallerstein, N., & Bernstein, E. (Summer 1994). Introduction to community empowerment, participatory education, and health. *Health Education Quarterly, 21*(2), 141-148.

Washington State Department of Health. (1996). *Assessment of local public health jurisdiction performance indicators.* Olympia, WA: WSDH.

Chapter 7

Aday, L. (1997). Vulnerable populations: A community-oriented perspective. *Family and Community Health, 19*(4), 1-18.

American Public Health Association & National Association of County Health Officials. (1991). *APEXPH: Assessment protocol for excellence in public health.* Washington, DC: NACHO.

American Public Health Association. (1991). *Healthy communities 2000: Model standards.* Washington, DC: APHA.

American Public Health Association & the Centers for Disease Control and Prevention. (1993). *The guide to implementing model standards: Eleven steps toward a healthy community.* Washington, DC., pp. 12-13.

Anderson, E.T., & McFarlane, J.M. (1996). *Community as partner.* Philadelphia: Lippincott.

Barriball, K.L., & Mackenzie, A. (1993). Measuring the impact of nursing interventions in the community. *Journal of Advanced Nursing, 18,* 401-407.

Butterfoss, F., Goodman, M., & Wandersman, A. (1993). Community coalitions for prevention and health promotion. *Health Education Research,* 8(3), 315-330.

Centers for Disease Control and Prevention (1996). Poverty and infant mortality: United States, 1988. *Morbidity and Mortality Weekly Report,* 44, 922-927.

Centers for Disease Control and Prevention (1998). *PATCH: Planned approach to community health.* Atlanta: CDC.

Conley, E. (1995). Public health nursing within core public health functions. *Journal of Public Health Management and Practice, 1*(3): 1-8.

DeFriese, G.H., & Crossland, C.L. (1995). Strategies, guidelines, policies and standards: The search for direction in community health promotion–criticisms from Canada. *Health Promotion International, 10*(1), 69-74.

Dever, G.E.A. (1997). *Improving outcomes in public health practice.* Gaithersburg, MD: Aspen.

Eng, E., & Parker, E. (1994). Measuring community competence in the Mississippi Delta: the interface between program evaluation and empowerment. *Health Education Quarterly, 21*(2), 199-200.

Fawcett, S.B., Paine-Andrews, A., & Francisco, V.T. (1995). Using empowerment theory in collaborative partnerships for community health and development. *American Journal of Community Psychology, 23*(5), 677-697.

Fitzpatrick, R., & White, D. (1997). Public participation in the evaluation of health care. *Health and Social Care in the Community, 5*(1), 3-10.

Flynn, B.C., & Dennis, L.I. (1996). Health promotion through healthy cities. In Stanhope, M., & Lancaster, J. (1997). *Community health nursing: promoting health of aggregates, families and individuals* (pp. 333-342). St. Louis: Mosby.

Flynn, B.C., Rider, M., & Ray, D.W. (1991). Healthy cities: The Indiana model of community development in public health. *Health Education Quarterly, 18*(3), 331-347.

Geltman, P.L., Meyers, A.F., Greenburg, J., & Zuckerman, B. (1996). Welfare reform and children's health. *Health Policy and Child Health, 3*(2), 1-5.

Gordon, R.L., Gerzoff, R.B., & Richards, T.B. (1997). Determinants of U.S. local health department expenditures, 1992 through 1993. *American Journal of Public Health, 87*(1), 91-95.

Green, L.W., & Kreuter, M.W. (1991). *Health promotion planning: An educational and environmental approach* (2nd ed.). Mountain View CA: Mayfield.

Hale, C.D., Arnold, F., & Travis, M.T. (1994). *Planning and evaluating health programs: A primer.* Albany, NY: Delmar.

Hancock, T. (1985). Beyond health care: From public health policy to healthy public policy. *Canadian Journal of Public Health, 76*(Suppl. 1), 9-11.

Hickman, P. (1997). Community partnerships. In Swanson, J., & Nies, M. (Eds.), *Community health nursing.* Philadelphia: WB Saunders.

Holloran, J.P., Ross, M.W., & Huffman, L. (1996). Training people with HIV disease for involvement in community planning process: Project LEAP, *Journal of the Association of Nurses in AIDS Care, 7*(6), 39-47.

Israel, B., Checkoway, B., Schulz, A., & Zimmerman, M. (1994). Health education and community empowerment: Conceptualizing and measuring perceptions of individual, organizational, and community control. *Health Education Quarterly, 21*(2), 149-170.

Kay, B.J., Share, D.A., Jones, K., Smith, M., Garcia, D., & Yeo, SA. (1991). Process, costs, and outcomes of community-based prenatal care for adolescents. *Medical Care, 29*(6), 531-542.

Link, B.G., & Phelan, J.C. (1996). Understanding sociodemographic differences in health: The role of fundamental social causes. *American Journal of Public Health.* 86:471-473.

May, K.M., Mendelson, C., & Ferketich, S. (1995). Community empowerment in rural health care. *Public Health Nursing, 12*(1), 25-30.

Miller, C.A., Moore, K.S., Richards, T.S., & Monk, J.D. (1994). A proposed method for assessing the performance of local public health functions and practices. *American Journal of Public Health, 84,* 1743-1749.

Richards, T.B., Rogers, J.J., Christenson, G.M., Miller, C.A., Gatewood, D.D., & Taylor, M.S. (1995). Assessing public health practice: application of ten core function measures of community health in six states. *American Journal of Preventive Medicine, 11*(Suppl. 2), 36-40.

Stanhope, M., & Knollmueller, R. (1997) *Public and community health nurse's consultant: A health promotion guide.* St. Louis: Mosby.

Stanhope, M., & Lancaster, J. (1996). *Community health nursing: promoting the health of aggregates, families and individuals* (4th ed.). St. Louis: Mosby.

Studnicki, I., Steverson, B., Blais, H.N., Goley, E., Richard, T.B., & Thornton, J.N. (1994). Analyzing organizational practices in local health departments. *Public Health Reports, 109*(4), 485-490.

Turnock, B.J. (1997). *Public health: What it is and how it works.* Gaithersburg, MD: Aspen.

United States Department of Health & Human Services. (1991). *Healthy people 2000: National health promotion and disease prevention objectives.* (DHHS No. 91-50212). Washington, DC: U.S. Government Printing Office.

United States Department of Health and Human Services. (1995). *Healthy people 2000: Midcourse review and 1995 revision.* Washington, DC: U.S. Government Printing Office.

United States Public Health Service. (1994). *For a healthy nation: Return on investments in public health.* Washington, DC: U.S. Government Printing Office.

Washington State Department of Health. (1996). *Assessment of local public health jurisdiction performance indicators.* Olympia, WA: WSDH.

Wells, J. (1996). The public and professional interface with priority setting in the National Health Service. *Health and Social Care in the Community, 4*(5), 255-263.

Winkelstein, W. (1992). Determinants of worldwide health. *American Journal of Public Health, 82*(7), 931-932.

Zerwekh, J.V. (1992). The practice of empowerment and coercion by expert public health nurses. *Image—The Journal of Nursing Scholarship, 24*(2), 101-105.

Chapter 8

Aday, L.A. (1993). *At risk in America: The health and health care needs of vulnerable populations in the United States.* San Francisco: Jossey-Bass.

Bushy, A. (1991). *Rural nursing* (Vols. 1-2). Newberry Park, CA: Sage.

Chick, V., & Phillips, B. (1993). Adequate access to post-hospital home health services: Differences between urban and rural areas. *The Journal of Rural Health, 9*(4), 262-269.

Coburn, A.F., & Mueller, K.J. (1995). Legislative and policy strategies for supporting rural health network development: Lessons from the 103rd. Congress. *The Journal of Rural Health, 11*(1), 22-31.

Comer, J., & Mueller, K. (1995). Access to health care: Urban-rural comparisons from a Midwestern agricultural state. *The Journal of Rural Health, 11*(2), 128-135.

Duncan, C.M. (Ed.). (1992). *Rural poverty in America.* New York: Auburn House.

Elnicki, D.M., Morris, D.K., & Shockor, W.T. (1995). Patient-perceived barriers to preventative health care among indigent, rural appalachian patients. *Archives of Internal Medicine, 155*(4), 421-424.

Hansen, M.M., & Resick, L.K. (1990). Health beliefs, health care, and rural Appalachian and non-Appalachian health professionals. *Family and Community Health, 13*(1), 1-10.

Stanhope, M., & Lancaster, J. (1996). *Community health nursing: Promoting the health of aggregates, families and individuals* (4th ed.). St. Louis: Mosby.

Strickland, W.J., & Strickland, D.L. (1995). Coping with the cost of care: An exploratory study of lower income minorities in the rural south. *Family and Community Health, 18*(2), 37-51.

Thobaden, M., & Weingard, M. (1983). Rural nursing. *Home Healthcare Nurse, 1*(2), 9-13.

Tripp-Reimer, T. (1982). Barriers to health care: Variations in interpretation of Appalachian and non-Appalachian health professionals. *Western Journal of Nursing Research, 4*(2), 179-191.

Tripp-Reimer, T., & Friedl, M.C. (1977). Appalachians: A neglected minority. *Nursing Clinics of North America, 12*(1), 41-54.

Winstead-Frya, P., Tiffany, J.C., & Shippee-Rice, R.V. (Eds.) (1992). *Rural health nursing.* New York: National League for Nursing Press.

Chapter 9

Austin, C.J., Johnson, J.A., & Palestrant, G.D. (1994). Information systems for human resources management. In Fottler, M.D., Hernandez, S.R., & Joiner, C.L. *Strategic management of human resources in health service organizations* (2nd. ed.). Albany, NY: Delmar.

Backer, T.E. (1995). Integrating behavioral and systems strategies to change clinical practice. *Journal on Quality Improvement, 21*(7), 351-354.

Boland, P. (1994). The challenge of documenting managed care cost savings and performance. *Managed Care Quarterly, 1*(4), 36-40.

Bower, K.A. (1992). The concept of case management. In *Case management by nurses* (pp. 3-9). Washington, DC: American Nurses Publishing.

Bower, K.A., & Falk, C.D. (1996). Case management as a response to quality, cost, and access imperatives. In Cohen, E.L. (Ed.), *Nurse case management in the 21st century* (Ch. 18). St. Louis: Mosby.

Cesta, T.G., Tahan, H.A., & Fink, L.K. (1998). *The case manager's survival guide: Winning strategies for clinical practice* (Ch. 1-4). St. Louis: Mosby.

Fox, P.D., & Fama, T. (1996). Managed care and chronic illness: An overview. In Fox, P.D., & Fama, T. (Eds.), *Managed care and chronic illness: Challenges and opportunities.* (pp. 3-5) Gaithersburg, MD: Aspen.

Gillies, D.A. (1994). *Nursing management: A systems approach.* Philadelphia: W.B. Saunders.

Gillies, R.R., Shortell, S.M., Anderson, D.A., Mitchell, J.B., & Morgan, K.L. (1993). Conceptualizing and measuring integration: Findings from the health systems integration study. *Hospital and Health Services Administration, 38*(4) 467-489.

Handy, C. (1994). *The age of paradox.* Boston, MA: Harvard Business School Press.

Hicks, L.L., Stallmeyer, J.M., & Coleman, J.R., (1993). Overview of managed care. In *Role of the nurse in managed care.* Washington, DC: American Nurses Publishing.

Institute for Health and Aging, University of California, San Francisco. (1996). *Chronic care in America: A 21st century challenge.* Princeton, NJ: The Robert Wood Johnson Foundation.

Lamb, G. (1995). Case management. *Annual Review of Nursing Research, 13,* 117-136.

May, C.A., Schraeder, C., & Britt, T. (1996). *Managed care and case management: Roles for professional nursing.* Washington, DC: American Nurses Publishing.

McGee, G.W. & Shewchuk, R.M. (1994). Managing a diverse work force. In Fottler, M.D., Hernandez, S.R., & Joiner, C.L. (Eds.), *Strategic management of human resources in health service organizations* (2nd. ed., Ch. 8). Albany, NY: Delmar.

McGlynn, E.A. (1996). Choosing chronic disease measures for HEDIS: Conceptual framework and review of seven clinical areas. In Fox, P.D., & Fama, T. (Eds.), *Managed care and chronic illness: Challenges and opportunities.* (pp. 18-57). Gaithersburg, MD: Aspen.

Mills, M.E., Romano, C.A., & Heller, B.R. (1996). *Information management in nursing and health care.* Springhouse, PA: Springhouse.

Mitchell, P.H., et al. (1997). Adverse outcomes and variations in organization of care delivery. *Medical Care, 35*(Suppl. 11), NS19-NS32.

O'Connor, S.J., & Proenca, E.J. (1994). Management of corporate culture. In Fottler, M.D., Hernandez, S.R., & Joiner, C.L. *Strategic management of human resources in health service organizations* (2nd. ed., Ch. 7). Albany, NY: Delmar.

Powell, S.K. (1996). *Nursing case management: A practical guide to success in managed care* (Ch. 5-6). Philadelphia: Lippincott.

Rohrer, J.E. (1996). *Planning for community-oriented health systems.* Washington, DC: American Public Health Association.

Sandy, L.G., & Gibson, R. (1996). Managed care and chronic care: Challenges and opportunities. In Fox, P.D., & Fama, T. (Eds.), *Managed care and chronic illness: Challenges and opportunities* (pp. 8-17). Gaithersburg, MD: Aspen.

Siefker, J.M., Garrett, M.B., Van Genderen, A., & Weis, M.J. (1997). *Fundamentals of case management* (Ch. 13-19, 25). St. Louis: Mosby.

Smith, H.L., & Fottler, M.D. (1994). Training and development. In Fottler, M.D., Hernandez, S.R., & Joiner, C.L. (Eds.), *Strategic management of human resources in health service organizations* (2nd. ed., Ch. 13). Albany, NY: Delmar.

Stanhope, M. (1996). Program planning. In Stanhope, M., & Lancaster, J. (Eds.) *Community health nursing: Promoting health of aggregates, families and individuals* (4th ed.). St. Louis: Mosby.

United States Department of Health and Human Services. (1991). *Healthy people 2000: National health promotion and disease prevention objectives.* (DHHS No. 91-50212). Washington, DC: U.S. Government Printing Office.

United States Department of Health and Human Services. (1995). *Healthy people 2000: Midcourse review and 1995 revision.* Washington, DC: U.S. Government Printing Office.

Valanis, B. (1992). *Epidemiology in nursing and health care* (2nd. ed.). Norwalk, CT: Appleton & Lange.

Walker, M.K., & Sebastian, J.G. (1997). Complementarity of advanced practice nursing roles in enhancing health outcomes of the chronically ill: Acute care nurse practitioners and nurse case managers. In Moorhead, S. & Huber, D.G. (Eds.), *Nursing roles: Evolving or recycled? Series on Nursing Administration.* Thousand Oaks, CA: Sage.

Winterbottom, C., Liska, D.W., & Obermaier, K.M. (1995). *State-level data book on health care access and financing.* Washington, DC: Urban Institute.

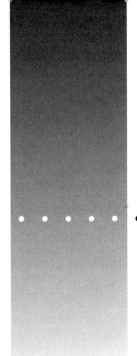

Index